Fire in the Valley

The TCM Diagnosis & Treatment of Vaginal Diseases

带下外阴阴道之病

Bob Flaws

BLUE POPPY PRESS

Published by:

BLUE POPPY PRESS, INC.
3450 Penrose Place, Suite 110
BOULDER, CO 80301

First Edition, June 1991
Second Edition, April 1994
Third Printing, January 1999

ISBN 0-936185-25-2 LC 91-72618

COPYRIGHT 1991 © BLUE POPPY PRESS

All rights reserved. No part of this book may be reproduced, stored in a retrieval system, transcribed in any form or by any means, electronic, mechanical, photocopy, recording, or any other means, or translated into any language without the prior written permission of the publisher.

The information in this book is given in good faith. However, the translators and the publishers cannot be held responsible for any error or omission. Nor can they be held in any way responsible for treatment given on the basis of information contained in this book. The publishers make this information available to English language readers for scholarly and research purposes only.

The publishers do not advocate nor endorse self-medication by laypersons. Chinese medicine is a professional medicine. Laypersons interested in availing themselves of the treatments described in this book should seek out a qualified professional practitioner of Chinese medicine.

COMP Designation: Compilation of functional translations using a standard translational terminology plus an original work

Printed at Bookcrafters in Chelsea, MI on recycled paper

10 9 8 7 6 5 4 3

Preface to the Second Edition

Dai xia is usually translated as abnormal vaginal discharge or leukorrhea. *Dai* means belt or girdle and refers to the *dai mai* or belt vessel. *Xia* means down or below. Traditionally, Chinese doctors specializing in gynecology were often called *dai xia yi* or *dai xia* doctors and *dai xia ke* or specialty in *dai xia* was a synonym for gynecology or problems below the belt. To this day, if one asks what constitutes traditional Chinese *fu ke* or gynecology, the answer is *jing dai chan hou* or menstrual complaints, *dai xia*, and pre and postpartum conditions. Zhang Zhong-qing's *Jin Gui Yao Lue (Essentials from the Golden Cabinet)* is the first Chinese medical classic to contain a chapter specifically devoted to gynecology. In that chapter, Zhang says,

> The 36 diseases that derive from vacuity and replete cold of the *dai mai* have a thousand variations. Therefore, it is necessary to carefully discriminate between yin and yang, vacuity and repletion, and tight bowstring [pulses] before applying acupuncture and medicinals in order to secure and save patients who may have the same disease but different pulses due to different causes. This rule must be remembered and should not be regarded with indifference.

As the above passage suggests, there are numerous varieties of female complaints associated with the *dai mai*. As a practitioner specializing in Chinese gynecology, I have spent considerable time going through the Chinese literature regarding *dai xia* and other related gynecological complaints. Although the English language literature on menstrual disorders is relatively complete, I feel that it is clinically incomplete regarding abnormal vaginal discharge, vaginitis, vulvitis, cervicitis, and vaginal itching. These are commonly encountered problems in clinical practice. Therefore, I would like to share my literary research on these problems with my fellow English-speaking practitioners.

Fire In The Valley

This is the first series of translations from the Chinese medical literature which I have undertaken essentially on my own. However, they could never have been completed without the support and assistance of my old friend Zhang Ting-liang who helped me find the characters I otherwise could not and clarified a number of colloquial expressions. These translations have been taken from a number of Chinese sources. These have been listed in the bibliography at the back of this book and the sources identified by title and author in the body of the text. Thanks are due to my Chinese herb teacher, Dr. Yu Min of the Yue Yang Hospital, Shanghai, for supplying me with a number of these books, especially those published in the last 2-3 years.

In preparing this revised edition, I have made the following changes in the text: 1) I tried, as far as possible, to use the terminology suggested by Nigel Wiseman in his *English-Chinese Chinese-English Dictionary of Chinese Medicine*, Changsha, 1995. I fully endorse Mr. Wiseman's arguments for and attempts to standardize our profession's technical terminology. For an iron-bound argument why such a linguistically accurate standard translational terminology is necessary within the English-speaking profession, please see Wiseman's essay on this subject at Paradigm Publications web page, www.paradigm-pubs.com.

2) I have added Pinyin in parentheses for all Chinese medicinals. 3) I have added English language translations for all Chinese medicinal formulas. 4) I have deleted some material which I feel had become dated and no longer expressed my point of view. And 5) I repaired some of the English which, in my attempts to remain as close to the Chinese as possible, was often stilted. Hopefully, these changes will make this book easier and more pleasant to use.

Since its initial writing, this book has become one of a several part series on Chinese gynecology. The other titles in this series include *A Handbook of Menstrual Diseases in Chinese Medicine; Path of Pregnancy, Vol. 1 & 2;* and *Fulfilling the Essence.* When taken together as a set, these books cover all areas of Chinese gynecology. For even more information on Chinese gynecology, Blue Poppy also has available a Postgraduate Certification Program in TCM Gynecology. This is comprised of professionally edited audiotapes of my lectures on Chinese gynecology plus hundreds of pages of otherwise unavailable translations from scores of premodern and contemporary Chinese gynecology texts and journal articles.

The identification of medicinal ingredients in this book is based on Bensky & Gamble's *Chinese Herbal Medicine: Materia Medica*; Hong-yen Hsu's *Oriental Materia Medica*; Cloudburst Press' *The Barefoot Doctor's Manual*; and Southern Materials Center's *Chinese Materia Medica*, Vol. 1-6. These identifications are made using a combination of Latinate pharmacological nomenclature plus Pinyin in parentheses. The first Latin word in each identification refers to the part of the plant or material used. Then the plant or animal's name follows given in the possessive case. Some of the formulas in this book specify the use of processed Chinese medicinals. Such processing increases the efficacy of Chinese medicinals when used for specific purposes. For further information on the use of processed Chinese medicinals, please see Philippe Sionneau's *Pao Zhi: An Introduction to the Used of Processed Chinese Medicinals* also available from Blue Poppy Press.

Bob Flaws
Boulder, CO
Oct. 1, 1998

Contents

v	Preface
1	Abnormal Vaginal Discharge *Dai Xia*
61	Vaginitis *Yin Dao Yan*
83	Vaginal Itch *Nu Yin Sau Yang Zheng*
97	Inflammatory Conditions of the External Genitalia *Wai Yin Bu Yan Zheng*
109	Herpes Genitalia *Sheng Qi Zhi Pao Zhen*
115	Genital Warts *Jian Rui Shi You*
119	Inflammatory Conditions of the Cervix *Gong Jing Yan Zheng*
135	Bibliography
139	Index

Abnormal Vaginal Discharge
Dai Xia

According to the authors of *Concise Traditional Gynecology*, women normally secrete a small amount of white, thin, slightly sticky, and odorless vaginal mucous between the ages of 14 and 50. Chinese medical theory associates this secretion with the so-called *tian gui* or heavenly water. This is indicated by the mention of the ages 14-50. Menarche is traditionally referred to as the arrival of the *tian gui* as is each period. Although some Chinese doctors consider the *tian gui* to be identical to the menstruate, others regard it as something related but different. Those that see the *tian gui* as different from the menstruate say that the *tian gui* precedes the arrival of the menses.

The *Nei Jing (Inner Classic)* states that the *tian gui* arrives at two times seven years of age when the kidney essence becomes exuberant. This essence becomes exuberant because of the accumulation of latter heaven or postnatal essence. Postnatal essence is transformed out of the finest essence of food and liquids absorbed by the spleen. The spleen and stomach are immature at birth and do not begin to function truly efficiently until around the age of six or seven. That means that until six or so, the postnatal essence is not exuberant even though the prenatal essence has the relatively pristine and unused quality of youth. The postnatal essence becomes exuberant only when the middle burner begins to mature, thus producing a superabundance daily of qi and blood beyond each day's immediate needs. This then is transformed into essence at night during sleep and is stored in the kidneys. By 14 in females, the source of postnatal essence is robust and fully functioning and the prenatal essence is still quite youthful and abundant. Since essence and blood share a common source, at 14 or thereabouts, females produce enough blood to fill the *chong mai* and *bao gong* or uterus full to overflowing. This monthly overflow of blood is the menstrual discharge.

However, not only do essence and blood share a common source but so do blood and fluids. Both blood and body fluids are part of the global *yin xue* or yin fluids and blood of the body. Both are moved and transformed by the qi, and both to move together. It is the heart (and lung qi since both together form the chest qi) which move the blood down the *bao mai* to the uterus each month in order to collect in the uterus and eventually brim over as the menstrual discharge. This qi which moves the blood downward also moves the body fluids downward at the same time since they are so closely related. This is why women's vaginal discharge increases prior to their menses. This is the *tian gui* or heavenly water which arrives or precedes the menstrual blood sent down from the heart.

This also explains why increases of vaginal discharge are normal at midcycle or ovulation and also during pregnancy. At midcycle, yin has reached its apogee. During and immediately after menstruation, blood and, therefore, also body fluids, tends to be vacuous or insufficient. From the end of menstruation till midcycle, blood and yin grows. This growth of body fluids along with blood manifests as increased vaginal fluids. Because yin is the root of yang and because yang is transformed from yin, at midcycle this abundance of yin gives rise to the growth of yang. Yang transforms yin and so this growth of yang moves and transforms vaginal yin fluids so that their level is more normal.

However, as described above, as blood moves down into the pelvis to accumulate in the uterus during the postovulatory or luteal phase, so do body fluids, thus resulting in more vaginal lubrication. Likewise, during pregnancy, there is the same focusing downward of blood on the uterus. This also results in the same downward movement of accompanying body fluids and increased vaginal discharge during pregnancy. Therefore, increased vaginal discharge or lubrication is considered normal, within certain parameters, at menarche (classically 14), midcycle, immediately premenstrually, and during pregnancy.

Dai Xia/Abnormal Vaginal Discharge

At seven times seven or 49-50 years of age, the *tian gui* becomes exhausted and the menses cease. This is because the *yang ming* or stomach and intestines begin to decline in function at around the age of 35 and the kidneys not long thereafter. In other words, postnatal production of acquired essence begins to fall off and the prenatal essence is not bolstered. By this time, prenatal essence is no longer pristine. Since every metabolic transformation uses a small bit of essence and source qi as substrate and catalyst respectively, by middle age, the kidneys' store is beginning to show signs of depletion. By 49 or 50, the woman's body no longer makes an excess of blood each month and cannot afford a monthly loss of blood and body fluids. Therefore, the body goes through a change whereby menstruation ceases in order to conserve more efficiently the kidneys' remaining essence. This change in life is an expression of a relative vacuity of yin, and since the vaginal fluids or mucous are part of the yin fluids, it too becomes scanty.

All this describes the production and fluctuations in normal vaginal secretions and fluids. These secretions and their variations are normal and healthy within these parameters. However, sometimes these fluids become excessive and mixed with other pathogenic factors and mechanisms. In that case, such abnormal vaginal discharges are categorized as *dai xia* in TCM. TCM subcategorizes *dai xia* into a number of different varieties. As mentioned in the preface, *dai xia* as a group accounts for one of the four major categories of traditional Chinese gynecological disease: *jing, dai, chan, hou/*or menstrual diseases, *dai xia*, pre, and postpartum diseases.

In modern TCM, the basic disease mechanisms of *dai xia* have to do with the downward flow or percolation of turbid dampness and the inhibition of the *ren* and *dai* vessels in controlling yin fluids. Although the *ren mai* is called the sea of yin, it carries primarily qi which then commands the blood and body fluids. Likewise, the *dai mai* carries mostly qi which restrains the downward percolation of fluids from the middle to the lower burner. Therefore, to say that *dai xia* is due to inhibition of the function of the *ren* and *dai* means that the movement and transportation of yin fluids by qi is dysfunctional or impaired.

Premodern Chinese Theory & Classification of *Dai Xia*

The premodern Chinese description of the causes of *dai xia* are more poetic and complex. According to Zhang Jing-yue, as quoted in Chen Lian-fang's Qing dynasty *Nu Ke Mi Jue Da Quan (The Complete Secrets of Success in Gynecology)*, there are six causes of *dai xia* all having to do in some way or another with the lifegate fire, one of Zhang Jing-yue's favorite topics. Zhang says that although there are different types of *dai xia*, they are all subsumed under the one large category of *dai xia* since all are in some way attributed to weakness of the *dai mai* which Zhang in turn relates to infirmity or lack of astringency of the lifegate. The implication here is that astringency of the *dai* is a function of the lifegate. This goes back to the fact that astringency is one of the five functions of qi and that the lifegate is identical to the moving qi between the kidneys, the prenatal source of all qi in the body. In particular, the qi of the *dai mai*, as an extraordinary vessel which absorbs repletion from the regular channels, is derived from the gallbladder, bladder, and stomach channels and all of these organs' warmth and function is founded upon the warming and steaming of the lifegate.

Zhang's first specific cause of *dai xia* has to do with the relationship of the heart to the lifegate. Zhang says that when the banner of the heart flutters, the lifegate responds and when the lifegate thus responds, it loses grasp of what it is supposed to hold. In other words, if the heart is upset by emotional fluctuations, this can cause an upward stirring of the ministerial fire like a militiaman who drops his work in order to answer a call to arms. The flaring upward of the lifegate results in a downward falling of that which the lifegate/*dai mai* should otherwise be holding and restraining, *i.e.*, body fluids.

Zhang's second disease mechanism resulting in *dai xia* is insatiable sexual desire. Zhang says that indulgence without regulation leads to slipperiness of the essence pathway and thus to failure of the lifegate. Sexual desire is a function of kidney yang. It is the source of arousal and excitement which makes us "hot and bothered". Orgasm is a crescendo of yang, a release of yang catalyzed and transformed from yin which travels up and

Dai Xia/Abnormal Vaginal Discharge

to the surface and is eventually discharged or lost from the body. Since it is the lifegate or kidney yang which holds the essence within the body, if yang is dissipated, the pathways of this essence may become slippery.

On the other hand, Zhang's third disease mechanism has to due with inability to orgasm or climax during intercourse. Chinese medicine says that men and women's ability to reach orgasm is like fire and water. Men are like fire. They ignite quickly but often burn out just as quickly. On the other hand, women are slow to boil. Zhang says that if a woman's sexual pleasure is interrupted halfway or without achieving orgasm, this causes a stoppage in the central pathway and this stoppage may cause counterflow. In turn, this counterflow may cause turbidity to drip down thus resulting in *dai xia*.

It was Zhang's opinion that these three mechanisms are responsible for the majority of cases of *dai xia* even though patients are reluctant to talk about these. He says that the turbidity which is associated with *dai xia* can be traced back to one of these three mechanisms in eight out of 10 cases. It was also Zhang's opinion that if the turbidity of *dai xia* is due to one of these three mechanisms and these three are not remedied and corrected, successful treatment cannot be achieved since internal medicine cannot triumph over erotic desire. Zhang Jing-yue says this is why *dai xia* is often recalcitrant to treatment.

Apart from the above three mechanisms, Zhang says the other three causes of *dai xia* are downward flow of dampness and heat, the lower source not securing due to vacuity cold, and weakness of astringency due to vacuity fall of the spleen and kidneys. It is these mechanisms which modern TCM authors mostly talk about and emphasize in their discussions of *dai xia*.

Xue Li-zhai, also quoted in *Nu Ke Mi Jue Da Quan*, felt that *dai xia* can be due to either the six external evils, the seven emotions, sex when drunk resulting in bedroom or sexual taxation, a preference for greasy, rich foods, injury due to overuse of drying medicinals, the downbearing and fall of yang qi due to vacuity and decline, or by the downbearing accumulation of dampness and phlegm. According to Xue, all these conditions should be treated by fortifying the spleen and promoting the upbearing of yang qi. This should be accomplished by different medicinals which each enter or gather in certain channels. For instance, *qing dai* or a greenish discharge should be treated by medicinals which enter the liver channel. Red *dai* should be treated by medicinals which enter the heart channel. White *dai* should be treated by medicinals which enter the lungs, yellow *dai*, the spleen, and black *dai*, the kidneys. We will speak more of these five colors of *dai* below.

The famous Qing dynasty gynecologist, Fu Qing-zhu, held that all kinds of excessive vaginal discharge are species of dampness. He emphasized failure of the *dai mai* in its controlling function. According to Fu Qing-zhu as quoted by Chen Liang-fang, it is known that the *dai mai* is connected with the *ren* and *du* vessels. It is the *ren* and *du* which are first affected and which then subsequently involve the *dai*.

The main function of the *dai mai* is to govern the uterus and the fetus. When the *dai mai* is debilitated, it finds it hard to maintain this control and connection. This then results in non-securing of the uterus and fetus and is, therefore, called tendency to miscarriage due to weakness of the *dai* and non-securing of the fetus due to injury of the *dai*. Such injury of the *dai* may be caused not only by injury of the qi due to fall or sudden sprain or strain but also by sexual indulgence and emotional fluctuations resulting from drinking wine. These activities may not cause physical pain or injury but result in insidious consumption of the qi, making it unable to transform the menstrual fluids. This then results in *dai xia*. Fu Qing-zhu goes on to say that, therefore, the victims of this condition are mostly married women, widows, and nuns but rarely virgins. Fu Qing-zhu adds that *dai xia* is natural when there is spleen qi vacuity, liver depression, invasion of damp qi, and oppression by hot qi.

Ye Tian-shi, another famous Qing dynasty internist also quoted by Chen Lian-fang, says that excessive vaginal discharge results in infertility and, therefore, merits immediate treatment. He then mentions that when the legendary Bian Que passed through Han Dan, he treated a noble lady there and, therefore, was famed as a *dai xia yi*.

According to Ye Tian-shi, if the discharge is red, heat has entered the small intestine. If the discharge is white, heat has entered the large intestine. The source of this heat can be traced back to the accumulation of damp heat in the *ren mai* which then infiltrates the bladder and lingers between the stomach and intestines. The liquid is secreted and tends to dribble down, hence the name *dai xia*. The volume in mild cases is moderate, but in severe cases it can be extremely heavy. If it is untreated, it will exhaust and dry the essence and blood causing emaciation of the flesh.

Again according to Ye Tian-shi, the primary emphasis in treating this condition should be to upbear yang and supplement yin in order to facilitate the spontaneous division of clear from turbid. Secondly, one should supplement the spleen and nourish the stomach in order to spontaneously eradicate damp heat. Patients should be encouraged to strengthen their resolve to abstain from greasy, rich foods, and original yang should be supplemented. Thus can an end be put to *dai xia*.

Classically, *dai xia* was subcategorized into the *wu dai* or five *dai*. Each of these is identified by a different color and each color corresponds to one of the five phases and, therefore, to one of the five viscera. Chen Lian-fang in *Nu Ke Mi Jue Da Quan* gives Fu Qing-zhu's descriptions of each of these five *dai* accompanied by his statement of their disease mechanisms, requisite treatment principles, and suggested internal treatment.

White *Dai, Bai Dai*

Fu Qing-zhu points out that so-called white vaginal discharge may happen to females at any time of the year and refers to the discharge of a white substance similar to saliva or clear nasal discharge. It is not voluntarily controllable and, in severe cases, it may smell offensively. Fu Qing-zhu says that *bai dai* is due to a predominance of dampness and decline of fire and liver depression and weakness of qi which damage the spleen and cause the qi of damp earth to pour downward. Spleen essence is not guarded and there is inability to transform the exuberant blood into the menstruate. On the contrary, this turns instead into a white, slippery substance which descends from the yin gate below and which is not controllable voluntarily.

In this case, the preferred therapeutic principles are to vigorously supplement the spleen and stomach qi assisted by medicinals for soothing the liver in order to free the flow of wind wood within earth. When earth qi surges by itself upward to heaven, spleen qi is fortified and damp qi is eliminated. This insures the termination of sufferings with *bai dai*. For these purposes, *Wen Dai Tang* is recommended.

Greenish *Dai, Qing Dai*

Fu Qing-zhu says that some females may have a greenish vaginal discharge. In some cases, this may be as green as mung bean soup, thick and mucousy, and may have an offensive odor. This is called *qing dai*. *Qing dai* is caused by damp heat in the liver channel. The liver pertains to wood and the color of wood is green. Hence, discharge as green as mung bean juice is due to disease of liver wood. Liver wood has a preference for water and mist, and dampness is the result of accumulation of water. At first sight, dampness is not what liver wood is averse to. How then can greenish discharge come into being? One should know that water is what the liver prefers but dampness is actually what liver wood detests the most. It is a fact that dampness pertains to the qi of earth. When what the liver favors is mixed with what the liver detests, there must be some disorder.

Since the preferences of the liver are ignored, liver qi is bound to become depressed. When this occurs, the qi needs to be upborne and dampness needs to be downborne since they impede each other and linger between the spaces of the middle burner. From there they find exit via the *dai mai* and yin orifice. The greenish color is the result of counteracting liver wood qi. When depression is mild, heat is not that prominent and, therefore, the color is merely greenish. But when depression is more extreme, heat is predominant and the color becomes dark green. It is believed that the treatment of greenish discharge is easier than that of the dark green variety. However, either can be eliminated by resolving the fire of liver wood and by disinhibiting bladder water. *Xiao Yao San* is recommended.

Yellow *Dai, Huang Dai*

Fu Qing-zhu says that yellowish vaginal discharge in females appears as a concentrated liquid like yellowish tea and may have a fetid odor. This is called *huang dai* or yellow *dai*. This yellowish discharge is due to damp heat in the *ren mai*. By its nature, the *ren mai* does not tolerate water, so how can dampness enter it and then be transformed into *huang dai*? To answer this, one should know that the *dai mai* bifurcates from the *ren mai* which then ascends vertically to connect with the gums and teeth. In between the teeth and gums there lies the source of a continuous spring of water which is connected by the *ren mai* to the lower (burner or source) for the purpose of participating in the process of transforming essence. Because of this connection, the *ren mai* is freed from the ill effects from the surrounding heat (which tends to waft up to the upper body) and all the saliva inside the mouth can be cultivated into essence which can then be stored in the kidneys.

However, when heat evils linger within the lower burner, mouth water fails to be transformed into essence. Instead, mouth water is transformed into dampness. This dampness actually belongs to the qi of earth and is the invasion of replete water. The heat belongs to the qi of fire and gives rise to replete wood. Water's color is black and fire's is red. When dampness becomes entangled with heat, it is impossible for this to be transformed into either red or black and the yellowish color is the outcome of this long term simmering process.

This condition is not due to water and fire but to dampness. Therefore it is not strange that treatment is ineffective if this situation is only thought of as damp heat of the spleen and treatment solely directed at the spleen. When this occurs, practitioners are not aware of the fact that true water and fire are surrounded by evils in the *dan tian* or the area of the former heaven source. These evils are entangled with the *ren mai* and its adjacent areas which are associated with conception of the fetus. Therefore, can treatment aimed solely at the spleen be effective? Rather, the correct method is to supplement vacuity of the *ren mai* and clear flaring fire from the kidneys. This condition can be remedied after a number of treatments and for it *Yi Huang Tang* is recommended.

Note: The *dan tian* and the source refer to the root of the body. Damp heat is a deviation of the qi of water and fire. Therefore the latter is a mixture of evils. This is like a mixture of pure silver, copper, and lead which does not, of course, constitute the righteous qi. Whenever true water and fire combine with evils, not only do they interpenetrate each other but they also change their own colors.

Black *Dai*, *Hei Dai*

According to Fu Qing-zhu, vaginal discharge in females which is dark in color, even as dark as black bean juice, and which has an offensive odor is called *hei dai* or black *dai*. Black *dai* is the outcome of extreme fire and heat. However, some may ask, since the color of fire is red, how can it turn into black which is the color of the extreme coldness of the lower (source, *i.e.*, kidney water)? When one asks such a question, it is because one is not aware of the resemblance of extreme fire to water. This is the false appearance of a true condition.

In this condition, there is always abdominal pain. There is also pain with urination and the genitalia are likely to be swollen. The facial complexion must be red and the patient is bound to become emaciated. Their appetite must be voracious, often accompanied by excessive thirst, and this makes one drink cold liquids which offer a modicum of relief. This is the outcome of exuberance of stomach fire and the subsequent mutual flaring or combination of stomach fire with lifegate, bladder, and triple heater fires. The process of drying out and turning into greyish discharge is the result of extreme fire and heat and is not due to moderate cold qi.

In this case, the victim may be manic. If not, kidney water and lung metal are given credit. In that case, their qi flows continuously and incessantly to moisten the heart and to support the stomach in an attempt to salvage the situation. The reason the discharge turns black is due to the accumulation of fire in the lower burner which then fails to flare upward. The best therapeutic approach is to drain fire and abate the great heat in order to eliminate dampness spontaneously. The formula *Li Huo Tang* is recommended.

Red *Dai*, *Chi Dai*

Again according to Fu Qing-zhu, if a woman has a reddish vaginal discharge which looks similar to blood and flows incessantly, this is called *chi dai* or red *dai*. Red *dai* is a damp condition and dampness pertains to the qi of earth which prefers the yellowish white color (to red). However, when a red substance is seen instead of a yellowish white colored substance, this is due to fire. Red is the color of fire. Therefore vaginal discharge caused by it looks red. The *dai mai* surrounds the waist and travels across the navel which is on the border of the area of extreme yin and in which fire is not supposed to be found. If a fire condition is found, does it mean that the fire of the lifegate is burning out through its connection with the *dai mai*? One should realize that the free flow of the *dai mai* is dependent upon the kidneys and the free flow of kidney qi is dependent upon the liver. In women, brooding and worry damage the spleen. This can be complicated by depression and anger damaging the liver. This then brews internally into depressive fire of the liver channel. Below, this overcomes spleen earth and spleen earth becomes unable to move and transform. Thus, lingering damp heat arises in the area governed by the *dai mai*.

One should also note that the failure of the liver to store blood allows the blood to seep into the *dai mai*. All this is due to damage of the spleen and inability of its transformative function. This permits damp heat to be released downward with qi and blood. The consequence of this is the appearance of a bloody looking substance but which is not actually blood. It is a fact that blood is indispensable to dampness. It is a grave mistake to attribute a red discharge to the fire of the heart. On the contrary, the treatment of this condition should be based on clearing liver fire and fortifying spleen qi. By doing so, just a few treatments can eradicate this problem. *Qing Gan Zhi Ling Tang* is recommended for this purpose.

Loose Turbidity, *Yin Zhuo*

Yin zhuo is a condition which was classically differentiated from *dai xia*. *Yin zhuo* is made up of two subcategories: *bai yin* or white looseness and *bai zhuo* or white turbidity. Like many Chinese disease names, *bai yin* is particularly difficult to translate. This *yin* means something loose and copious and also moral looseness. One Chinese translator I queried on this suggested erotic turbidity as the translation of the larger category. In Chinese, this word *yin* seems to be a *double entendre* and I have chosen the English word loose which carries these same two meanings.

Chen Lian-fang gives Zhang Jing-yue's discrimination of these two conditions. According to Zhang, the difference between *bai yin* and *bai zhuo* lies in the fact that white turbidity is excreted from the uterus and is a surplus from that organ. Whereas, white looseness is excreted from the bladder and results from turbid water. The kidneys are the source of *bai zhuo* since the kidneys and bladder have a mutual exterior/interior relationship. It should be remembered that vaginal discharge is mostly due to vacuity of the spleen and kidneys and *yin zhuo* is more due to damp heat of the bladder. This the general distinction between these two disease categories.

White Looseness, *Bai Yin*

Chen next gives Ye Tian-shi's discussion of *bai yin*. According to Ye Tian-shi, if *bai yin* accompanies urination and is turbid like rice washing water, this is due to the penetration of the bladder by turbid qi from the stomach. It is also classified as a species of *dai*. *Yi Zhi Tang* is the recommended formula.

White Turbidity, *Bai Zhuo*

Ye Tian-shi says that when white turbidity dribbles down and is sticky, chilly, and clear in appearance or if it trickles down after urination, this is due to vacuity detriment of the lower source qi. Because of inability to secure and astringe, this gives rise to slipperiness. This also should be classified as a species of *dai*. The formula *Fen Qing Yin* is suggested.

The above discrimination of *bai zhuo, bai yin,* and *bai dai* is essentially the same as that given by Mo Qian, also called Mi Zhai, of the Ming dynasty in his *Wan Min Fu Ren Ke (Gynecology for 10,000 People)*. Mo Qian says that these three conditions are frequently encountered in women and that, although they are not exactly the same, their treatment is not necessarily different. *Bai dai* may sometimes be normal and sometimes stream out. It may be chilly and clear or thick like glue. It is due to vacuity detriment of the lower source and one should use the treatment method of stopping *dai* if it has been going on for a long time without ceasing. *Bai zhuo* consists of a turbid discharge which follows or occurs at the same time as urination. It may be turbid like swill and is due to turbid qi from the stomach and middle oozing or seeping into the bladder.

Formulas for the Treatment of *Dai Xia*

The 29th chapter of *Nu Ke Mi Jue Da Quan* is devoted to describing the ingredients of the formulas for *dai xia* recommended by Fu Qing-zhu and Zhang Jing-yue above.

1. Qi-boosting Formulas

A. *Shou Pi Jian* (Long-life Spleen Decoction)

This formula was created by Zhang Jing-yue. It treats spleen vacuity not able to contain the blood in women without fire who have flooding and leaking, *i.e.*, uterine bleeding and other such conditions.

Rhizoma Atractylodis Macrocephalae (*Bai Zhu*), 6-9g
Semen Nelumbinis Nuciferae (*Lian Zi*), 20 pcs, remove the heart and stir-fry
Radix Panacis Ginseng (*Ren Shen*), 3-6g
mix-fried Radix Glycyrrhizae (*Gan Cao*), 3g
Semen Zizyphi Spinosae (*Suan Zao Ren*), 4.5g
Radix Angelicae Sinensis (*Dang Gui*), 6g
Radix Dioscoreae Oppositae (*Shan Yao*), 6g
processed Radix Polygalae Tenuifoliae (*Yuan Zhi*), 1-1.5g
blast-fried Rhizoma Zingiberis (*Pao Jiang*), 3-9g

If one has a slippery, uncontainable discharge, add 3 grams of vinegar-fried Concha Meretricis (*Hai Ge Ke*). If one's qi is very vacuous, add 6-9 grams of Radix Astragali Membranacei (*Huang Qi*). If one's central qi has fallen, add 1.5-1.7 grams of Rhizoma Cimicifugae (*Sheng Ma*). It is also possible to add Radix Angelicae Dahuricae (*Bai Zhi*).

B. *Huan Dai Tang* (Moderate *Dai* Decoction)

This formula was created by Fu Qing-zhu and is for supplementing the spleen and coursing the liver. It is effective for treating *dai xia*.

earth stir-fried Rhizoma Atractylodis Macrocephalae (*Bai Zhu*), 30g
stir-fried Radix Dioscoreae Oppositae (*Shan Yao*), 30g
Radix Panacis Ginseng (*Ren Shen*), 6g
wine stir-fried Radix Albus Paeoniae Lactiflorae (*Bai Shao*), 15g
wine stir-fried Semen Plantaginis (*Che Qian Zi*), 9g
stir-fried Rhizoma Atractylodis (*Cang Zhu*), 9g
Radix Glycyrrhizae (*Gan Cao*), 3g
Pericarpium Citri Reticulatae (*Chen Pi*), 1.5g
blackened Herba Schizonepetae Tenuifoliae (*Jing Jie*), 1.5g
Radix Bupleuri (*Chai Hu*), 1.7g

C. *Bu Zhong Yi Qi Tang* (Supplement the Center & Boost the Qi Decoction)

Radix Panacis Ginseng (*Ren Shen*), 4.5g

mix-fried Radix Astragali Membranacei (*Huang Qi*), 4.5g
mix-fried Rhizoma Atractylodis Macrocephalae (*Bai Zhu*), 4.5g
mix-fried Radix Glycyrrhizae (*Gan Cao*), 4.5g
Radix Angelicae Sinensis (*Dang Gui*), 3g
Pericarpium Citri Reticulatae (*Chen Pi*), 1.5g
Rhizoma Cimicifugae (*Sheng Ma*), 1.2g
Radix Bupleuri (*Chai Hu*), 1.2g
uncooked Rhizoma Zingiberis (*Sheng Jiang*), 3 slices
Fructus Zizyphi Jujubae (*Da Zao*), 2 pcs

D. *Si Jun Zi Tang* (Four Gentlemen Decoction)

Radix Panacis Ginseng (*Ren Shen*), 9g
Rhizoma Atractylodis Macrocephalae (*Bai Zhu*), 9g
Sclerotium Poriae Cocos (*Fu Ling*), 9g
Radix Glycyrrhizae (*Gan Cao*), 3g

E. *Liu Jun Zi Tang* (Six Gentlemen Decoction)

To *Si Jun Zi Tang* above add:

Rhizoma Pinelliae Ternatae (*Ban Xia*), 4.5g
Pericarpium Citri Reticulatae (*Chen Pi*), 4.5g

2. Warming the Lower (Burner/Source) Formulas

A. *Yi Zhi Tang* (Boost the Intelligence Decoction)

This formula treats *bai yin* or white looseness.

Pericarpium Citri Reticulatae (*Chen Pi*), 6g
Sclerotium Poriae Cocos (*Fu Ling*), 6g
mix-fried Rhizoma Atractylodis Macrocephalae (*Bai Zhu*), 6g
mix-fried Radix Glycyrrhizae (*Gan Cao*), 6g
stir-fried Rhizoma Atractylodis (*Cang Zhu*), 6g
Semen Coicis Lachryma-jobi (*Yi Yi Ren*), 3g
Radix Bupleuri (*Chai Hu*), 3g

Rhizoma Cimicifugae (*Sheng Ma*), 1.5g

B. *Fen Qing Yin* (Divide the Clear Drink)

This formula treats *bai zhuo* or white turbidity.

Rhizoma Dioscoreae Hypoglaucae (*Bei Xie*), 4.5g
Saltwater stir-fried Semen Coicis Lachryma-jobi (*Yi Yi Ren*), 4.5g
Radix Linderae Strychnifoliae (*Wu Yao*), 4.5g
Rhizoma Acori Graminei (*Shi Chang Pu*), 4.5g
Sclerotium Poriae Cocos (*Fu Ling*), 4.5g
stir-fried Fructus Citri Aurantii (*Zhi Ke*), 3g
mix-fried Radix Glycyrrhizae (*Gan Cao*), 3g

C. *Bai Shao Yao San* (White Peony Powder)

This formula created by Hai Zang treats like magic women's red and white *dai xia* with aching and pain in the navel and abdomen.

stir-fried Radix Albus Paeoniae Lactiflorae (*Bai Shao*), 30g
blast-fried Radix Zingiberis (*Pao Jiang*), 15g

Grind the above into fine powder. Each time take 9 grams followed by rice soup.

3. Enriching Yin Formulas

A. *Liu Wei Di Huang Wan* (Six Flavors Rehmannia Pills)

This formula treats kidney water depletion and detriment, dribbling, non-free flowing urination, and that sort of condition.

cooked Radix Rehmanniae (*Shu Di*), 9g
Fructus Corni Officinalis (*Shan Zhu Yu*), 4.5g
stir-fried Radix Dioscoreae Oppositae (*Shan Yao*), 4.5g
Cortex Radicis Moutan (*Dan Pi*), 3g

Rhizoma Alismatis (*Ze Xie*), 3g
Sclerotium Poriae Cocos (*Fu Ling*), 3g

B. *Bao Yin Jian* (Protect Yin Decoction)

This formula was created by Zhang Jing-yue. It treats blood flooding (profuse uterine bleeding) and bloody strangury in patients with yin vacuity and internal heat and bleeding conditions.

uncooked Radix Rehmanniae (*Sheng Di*), 6g
cooked Radix Rehmanniae (*Shu Di*), 6g
Radix Albus Paeoniae Lactiflorae (*Bai Shao*), 6g
Radix Dipsaci (*Xu Duan*), 4.5g
Radix Scutellariae Baicalensis (*Huang Qin*), 4.5g
Cortex Phellodendri (*Huang Bai*), 4.5g
Radix Glycyrrhizae (*Gan Cao*), 3g

If the blood is very hot, add 3 grams of Rhizoma Coptidis Chinensis (*Huang Lian*). If the blood is vacuous and stagnant, add 3-6 grams of Radix Angelicae Sinensis (*Dang Gui*). If there is blood discharge and slipperiness, add 3-6 grams of Radix Sanguisorbae (*Di Yu*) or 1-2 pieces of Fructus Pruni Mume (*Wiu Mei*) or 3 grams of *Bai Yao Qian* (identification unknown, possible typographical error in the original); Concha Meretricis (*Hai Ge Ke*) is also okay. For stagnant qi and pain, delete the cooked Rehmannia and add Pericarpium Citri Reticulatae (*Chen Pi*), Pericarpium Citri Reticulatae Viride (*Qing Pi*), Cortex Radicis Moutan (*Dan Pi*), and Rhizoma Cyperi Rotundi (*Xiang Fu*).

4. Securing the Root Formulas

A. *Mi Yuan Jian* (Secrete the Source Decoction)

This formula of Zhang Jing-yue's treats seminal emission and the *dai zhuo* category of diseases.

processed Radix Polygalae Tenuifoliae (*Yuan Zhi*), 1.8g
stir-fried Radix Dioscoreae Oppositae (*Shan Yao*), 6g
Semen Euryalis Ferocis (*Qian Shi*), 6g
stir-fried Semen Zizyphi Spinosae (*Suan Zao Ren*), 6g
stir-fried Rhizoma Atractylodis Macrocephalae (*Bai Zhu*), 4.5g Sclerotium Poriae Cocos (*Fu Ling*), 4.5g
mix-fried Radix Glycyrrhizae (*Gan Cao*), 3g
Radix Panacis Ginseng (*Ren Shen*), 3-6g
Fructus Schisandrae Chinensis (*Wu Wei Zi*), 14 pcs
Fructus Rosae Laevigatae (*Jin Ying Zi*), 6g

This formula treats enduring looseness without fire or pain. If there is emission, use this combination. If the patient still has fire and feels hot, add Radix Sophorae Flavescentis (*Ku Shen*), 3-6g.

B. *Suo Jing Wan* (Draw Back the Essence Pills)

This formula treats *bai zhuo* and polyuria.

Fructus Psoraleae Corylifoliae (*Bu Gu Zhi*)
Sodium Chloride (*Shi Yan*)
Sclerotium Poriae Cocos (*Fu Ling*)
Fructus Schisandrae Chinensis (*Wu Wei Zi*)

For one packet, use five times as many of the seeds as the other ingredients which should be equally divided. Grind the above into powder and make pills the size of Semen Dryandrae Cordata (tung tree seeds) by binding with wine. Take 30 pills each time on an empty stomach and wash down with warm wine.

C. *Jin Ying Gao* (Rosa Laevigata Paste)

This formula treats vacuity taxation, seminal emission, and *bai zhuo* and is extremely effective.

Fructus Rosae Laevigatae (*Jin Ying Zi*) (remove the pit and boil the juice until stewed down into a paste)
Radix Panacis Ginseng (*Ren Shen*)
Ootheca Mantidis (*Sang Piao Xiao*)
Radix Dioscoreae Oppositae (*Shan Yao*), 60g each
Cortex Eucommiae Ulmoidis (*Du Zhong*)
Fructus Alpiniae Oxyphyllae (*Yi Zhi Ren*), 30g each
Semen Coicis Lachryma-jobi (*Yi Yi Ren*)
Fructus Evodiae Rutecarpae (*Wu Zhu Yu*)
Semen Euryalis Fertocis (*Qian Shi*)
Fructus Lycii Chinensis (*Gou Qi Zi*), 120g each
Sodium Chloride (*Shi Yan*), 9g

Decoct the above in water two times. Remove the dregs and stew into a paste. Take on an empty stomach with 3-4 spoonfuls of pure, boiled water.

D. *Wei Xi Wan* (Mighty Joy Pills)

This harmonizing formula treats source yang vacuity seminal emission in men and *bai zhuo* in women with enduring desertion of the sea of blood, excessive *dai*, dream emission, and that category of diseases.

Take 120 grams of Sclerotium Poriae Cocos (*Fu Ling*). Do not use Sclerotium Polypori Umbellati (*Zhu Ling*). Remove the skin and cut into pieces 7.5 grams apiece. Put in a porcelain container and boil for 20 or more minutes. Remove the Poria and sun dry. Then take the Poria and powder it. Mix this powder with 120 grams of yellow wax and make pills the size of *tan* seeds. Take on an empty stomach after producing profuse saliva. Swallow very slowly. This formula is effective for clearing the urine.

E. *Gu Yin Jian* (Secure Yin Decoction)

This formula treats yin vacuity slippery discharge, turbidity, and involuntary pouring or precipitation (like rain pouring down) and when the menstrual discharge causes vacuity loss of astringency and other such conditions.

Radix Panacis Ginseng (*Ren Shen*) use whatever amount one wants
cooked Radix Rehmanniae (*Shu Di*), 6-15g
stir-fried Radix Dioscoreae Oppositae (*Shan Yao*), 6g
Fructus Evodiae Rutecarpae (*Wu Zhu Yu*), 4.5g
processed Radix Polygalae Tenuifoliae (*Yuan Zhi*),   2g
mix-fried Radix Glycyrrhizae (*Gan Cao*), 3-6g
Fructus Schisandrae Chinensis (*Wu Wei Zi*), 14 pcs
stir-fried till fragrant Semen Cuscutae Chinensis (*Tu Si Zi*), 6-9g

If there is extreme vacuity and involuntary emission, add 6-9 grams of the flesh of Fructus Rosae Laevigatae (*Jin Ying Zi*) or three grams of vinegar stir-fried Concha Meretricis (*Hai Ge Ke*) or two pieces of Fructus Pruni Mume (*Wu Mei*). For lack of astringency of the menstrual blood, add six grams of Radix Dipsaci (*Chuan Duan*). If the blood does not return to the channels, add 6-9 grams of Radix Angelicae Sinensis (*Dang Gui*). If the qi has fallen and is not astringing or securing, add three grams of Rhizoma Cimicifugae (*Sheng Ma*).

5. Heat-discharging Formulas

A. *Qing Xin Lian Zi Yin* (Clear the Heart Lotus Seed Drink)

This formula treats heat in the qi division with dry mouth, oral thirst, urination accompanied by pouring of turbidity, and similar conditions.

Radix Scutellariae Baicalensis (*Huang Qin*)
Tuber Ophiopogonis Japonici (*Mai Dong*)
Cortex Radicis Lycii Chinensis (*Di Gu Pi*)
Semen Plantaginis (*Che Qian Zi*), 4.5g each

Dai Xia/Abnormal Vaginal Discharge

Radix Panacis Ginseng (*Ren Shen*)
Radix Astragali Membranacei (*Huang Qi*)
Semen Nelumbinis Nuciferae (*Lian Zi*)
Radix Bupleuri (*Chai Hu*)
Sclerotium Poriae Cocos (*Fu Ling*), 3g each

B. *Long Dan Xie Gan Tang* (Gentiana Drain the Liver Decoction)[1]

This formula treats damp heat in the liver channel with red urination and other such categories of disease.

wine stir-fried Radix Gentianae Scabrae (*Long Dan Cao*)
Radix Panacis Ginseng (*Ren Shen*)
Tuber Asparagi Cochinensis (*Tian Men Dong*)
Tuber Ophiopogonis Japonici (*Mai Dong*)
Radix Glycyrrhizae (*Gan Cao*)
Rhizoma Coptidis Chinensis (*Huang Lian*)
Fructus Gardeniae Jasminoidis (*Zhi Zi*)
Rhizoma Anemarrhenae Aspheloidis (*Zhi Mu*), 1.5g each
Radix Scutellariae Baicalensis (*Huang Qin*), 2g
Radix Bupleuri (*Chai Hu*), 3g
Fructus Schisandrae Chinensis (*Wu Wei Zi*), 1g

C. *Yi Huang Tang* (Change Yellow Decoction)

This treats yellow *dai* and clears kidney fire.

stir-fried Radix Dioscoreae Oppositae (*Shan Yao*), 30g
Semen Euryalis Ferocis (*Qian Shi*), 30g
saltwater stir-fried Cortex Phellodendri (*Huang Bai*), 30g
wine stir-fried Semen Plantaginis (*Che Qian Zi*), 60g
Semen Gingkonis Bilobae (*Yin Guo*), 10 pcs, crushed

---

[1] Readers should note that this is not the usual *Long Dan Xie Gan Tang*. Either the ingredients are erroneous in the source text, or this is a different version of the formula of this name.

D. *Li Huo Tang* (Disinhibit Fire Decoction)

This formula by Fu Qing-zhu treats *hei dai* or black *dai*.

Radix Et Rhizoma Rhei (*Da Huang*), 9g
earth stir-fried Rhizoma Atractylodis Macrocephalae (*Bai Zhu*), 15g
Sclerotium Poriae Cocos (*Fu Ling*), 9g
wine stir-fried Semen Plantaginis (*Che Qian Zi*), 9g
Rhizoma Coptidis Chinensis (*Huang Lian*), 3g
blackened Fructus Gardeniae Jasminoidis (*Zhi Zi*), 9g
Rhizoma Anemarrhenae Aspheloidis (*Zhi Mu*), 6g
Semen Vaccariae Segetalis (*Wang Bu Liu Xing*), 9g
calcined Gypsum Fibrosum (*Shi Gao*), 15g
Herba Artemisiae Anomalae (*Liu Ji Nu*), 9g

E. *Qing Gan Zhi Lin Tang* (Clear the Liver & Stop Strangury Decoction)

This formula, also by Fu Qing-zhu, treats *chi* or red *dai*. It clears the liver and supports the spleen.

wine stir-fried Radix Albus Paeoniae Lactiflorae (*Bai Shao*), 30g
wine stir-fried Radix Angelicae Sinensis (*Dang Gui*), 30g
wine stir-fried uncooked Radix Rehmanniae (*Sheng Di*), 15g
Gelatinum Corii Asini (*E Jiao*), 9g, stir-fried in wheat flour
Cortex Radicis Moutan (*Dan Pi*), 9g
Cortex Phellodendri (*Huang Bai*), 6g
Radix Achyranthis Bidentatae (*Niu Xi*), 6g
wine stir-fried Rhizoma Cyperi Rotundi (*Xiang Fu*), 3g
Fructus Zizyphi Jujubae (*Da Zao*), 10 pcs
small Semen Glycinis Hispidae (*Xiao Hei Dou*), 30g

6. Dampness-disinhibiting Formulas

A. *Wu Ling San* (Five [Ingredients] Poria Powder)

This formula is from Zhang Zhong-qing. It treats inhibition of the urination with thirst, dribbling and dripping with pain, and damp heat in the lower part of the body.

Rhizoma Atractylodis Macrocephalae (*Bai Zhu*)
Sclerotium Poriae Cocos (*Fu Ling*)
Sclerotium Polypori Umbellati (*Zhu Ling*), 22.5g each
Cortex Cinnamomi Cassiae (*Rou Gui*), 15g
Rhizoma Alismatis (*Ze Xie*), 37.5 g

Grind the above ingredients and take six grams each time chased down with white soup (*i.e.*, dilute rice soup). Nowadays, the numbers of each ingredient are reduced and the herbs decocted in water and drunk.

B. *Si Ling San* (Four [Ingredients] Poria Powder)

Remove Cortex Cinnamomi from the preceding *Wu Ling San*.

C. *Hua Shi San* (Transform Dampness Powder)

This formula treats hot urinary strangury or dribbling.

Talcum (*Hua Shi*), 1.5g
Medulla Tetrapanacis Papyriferi (*Deng Xin Cao*), 1.1g
Semen Plantaginis (*Che Qian Zi*), 1.1g
Semen Abutilonis Seu Malvae (*Dong Kui Zi*), 1.1g

Grind the above medicinals and take with water.

7. Depression-opening Formulas

A. *Jia Jian Xiao Yao San* (Modified Rambling Powder)

This formula treats *qing dai* or greenish vaginal discharge. It resolves liver depression and eliminates damp heat.

Sclerotium Poriae Cocos (*Fu Ling*), 15g
wine stir-fried Radix Albus Paeoniae Lactiflorae (*Bai Shao*), 15g Radix Glycyrrhizae (*Gan Cao*), 15g
Radix Bupleuri (*Chai Hu*), 3g
Pericarpium Citri Reticulatae (*Chen Pi*), 3g
Herba Artemisiae Capillaris (*Yin Chen Hao*), 9g
blackened Fructus Gardeniae Jasminoidis (*Zhi Zi*), 9g

B. *Jia Wei Xiao Yao San* (Added Flavors Rambling Powder)

This harmonizing formula is a version of *Xiao Yao San* created by Zhang Jing-yue. It treats liver depression qi stagnation, cold and hot cough, and menstrual irregularity.

cooked Radix Rehmanniae (*Shu Di*)
Radix Angelicae Sinensis (*Dang Gui*)
Fructus Zizyphi Jujubae (*Da Zao*)
Radix Albus Paeoniae Lactiflorae (*Bai Shao*)
Sclerotium Pararadicis Poriae Cocos (*Fu Shen*)
mix-fried Radix Glycyrrhizae (*Gan Cao*)
Radix Polygalae Tenuifoliae (*Yuan Zhi*)
Pericarpium Citri Reticulatae (*Chen Pi*)

Decoct in water and take. No dosages are given. If there is qi vacuity, add Radix Panacis Ginseng (*Ren Shen*). If the menses are behind schedule, *i.e.*, late, and there is sluggishness and pain, add wine stir-fried Rhizoma Cyperi Rotundi (*Xiang Fu*).

C. *Gui Pi Tang* (Restore the Spleen Decoction)

This formula treats heart-spleen depression and binding and menstrual irregularity.[2]

Radix Panacis Ginseng (*Ren Shen*), 9g
Radix Astragali Membranacei (*Huang Qi*), 12g
Radix Angelicae Sinensis (*Dang Gui*), 9g
Arillus Euphoriae Longanae (*Long Yan Rou*), 9gt
Rhizoma Atractylodis Macrocephalae (*Bai Zhu*), 9g
Radix Auklandiae Lappae (*Mu Xiang*), 6g
Sclerotium Poriae Cocos (*Fu Ling*), 9g
Radix Polygalae Tenuifoliae (*Yuan Zhi*), 9g
Semen Zizyphi Spinosae (*Suan Zao Ren*), 12g
mix-fried Radix Glycyrrhizae (*Gan Cao*), 6g
uncooked Rhizoma Zingiberis (*Sheng Jiang*), 3 slices
Fructus Zizyphi Jujubae (*Da Zao*), 5-7 pcs

8. Qi, Blood & Yang Supplementing Formulas

A. *Ba Zhen Tang* (Eight Pearls Decoction)

This formula treats (the ill after effects of) excessive bleeding during labor and qi and blood depletion and decline. It is comprised of *Si Jun Zi Tang* described above and *Si Wu Tang* (Four Materials Decoction).

Radix Panacis Ginseng (*Ren Shen*), 9g
cooked Radix Rehmanniae (*Shu Di*), 12g
Rhizoma Atractylodis Macrocephalae (*Bai Zhu*), 9g
Radix Angelicae Sinensis (*Dang Gui*), 9g
Radix Albus Paeoniae Lactiflorae (*Bai Shao*), 9g
Radix Ligustici Wallichii (*Chuan Xiong*), 6g
Sclerotium Poriae Cocos (*Fu Ling*), 9g

---

[2] This formula is more usually indicated for heart blood-spleen qi vacuity.

mix-fried Radix Glycyrrhizae (*Gan Cao*), 6g

B. *Ba Zhen Yi Mu Wan* (Eight Pearls Leonurus Pills)

This formula treats qi and blood vacuity with diminished appetite, bent body, low back weakness, and abdominal distention with possible fever and chills. The menses are irregular and there may be red and white *dai xia*. This formula consists of *Ba Zhen Tang* above plus 120 grams of Herba Leonuri Heterophyllae (*Yi Mu Cao*).[3]

C. *Shi Quan Da Bu Tang* (Ten [Ingredients] Completely & Greatly Supplementing Decoction)

This formula is composed of *Ba Zhen Tang* plus Radix Astragali Membranacei (*Huang Qi*) and Cortex Cinnamomi Cassiae (*Rou Gui*).

Addendum: To the above list of formulas given in *Nu Ke Mi Jue Da Quan*, I would like to append the prescription Mo Qian gives for *bai yin, bai zhuo, bai dai*. It is *Jia Wei Er Chen Tang* (Added Flavors Two Aged [Ingredients] Decoction).

Pericarpium Citri Reticulatae (*Chen Pi*)
Rhizoma Pinelliae Ternatae (*Ban Xia*)
Sclerotium Poriae Cocos (*Fu Ling*)
Rhizoma Atractylodis Macrocephalae (*Bai Zhu*)
Rhizoma Atractylodis (*Cang Zhu*)
saltwater stir-fried Semen Coicis Lachryma-jobi (*Yi Yi Ren*), 3g each
Folium Artemisiae Argyii (*Ai Ye*), 1.5g
Rhizoma Cimicifugae (*Sheng Ma*)
Radix Bupleuri (*Chai Hu*), 2g each
uncooked Rhizoma Zingiberis (*Sheng Jiang*), 1 slice

---

[3] This amount of Leonurus is when this formula is made into pills. As a decoction, it may be prescribed at the standard 9 grams.

Tian Jian-lai, "On *Dai Xia*"

Tian Jian-lai was a Qing dynasty doctor living during the 18th century. He is the author of *Ling Yan Liang Fang Hui Bian (A Collection of Miraculously Effective Formulas)*. This book is mainly a compendium of formulas arranged by traditional Chinese disease categories. Preceding each category, Tian gives a brief discussion of the disease causes, mechanisms, and therapeutic principles involved. Although Tian's emphasis is on empirically efficacious prescriptions, he has arranged these according to pattern discrimination categorization. Thus one can see the beginnings of TCM methodology in Tian's presentation.

Abnormal vaginal discharge in women may be caused by the six excessive or wanton (evils) or the seven passions. It may be caused by drunkenness and sexual taxation or fatty meats and rich grains with thick flavors (*i.e.*, damp, greasy properties). Or it may be caused by excessive dosing with drying drugs. These may result in spleen- stomach vacuity damage. Yang qi may fall or become bogged down, or phlegm dampness may pour downward, seeping towards the bladder and becoming established there. The treatment method mainly ought to fortify the spleen and stomach and upbear the qi and blood.

Ancient formulas were named for the white type (of *dai xia*) having to do with qi and cold and the red type (having to do with) blood and heat. The main reason for (*dai xia*) is lack of free flow. (In Zhu) Dan-xi's opinion, this mostly has to do with the transformation of blood and establishment of phlegm. If the menstrual water comes like phlegm from the uterus, surely the low back and knees will feel faint. (In this case, it is) appropriate to simultaneously treat phlegm. Or the menstrual water may arrive purple and black. The lower abdomen will necessarily be chilly and the patient will get pleasure from eating hot things. It is appropriate to treat this with acrid, warm medicinals. If stomach turbidity sinks downward, one must supplement the stomach, upbear and lift. If there is damp heat, one must clear (heat), cool (the blood), resolve (toxins), and disinhibit (dampness). If there is vacuity detriment, one must simultaneously supplement the qi and the blood. Therefore, just as in dribbling and dripping (disorders), one cannot (simply) use stopping (*dai*) and astringing (the essence) medicinals.

Sheng Yang Sheng Shi Tang (Upbear Yang & Overcome Dampness Decoction)[4]

Radix Bupleuri (*Chai Hu*)
Radix Et Rhizoma Notopterygii (*Qiang Huo*)
Rhizoma Atractylodis (*Cang Zhu*)
Radix Astragali Membranacei (*Huang Qi*)
Radix Ledebouriellae Divaricatae (*Fang Feng*)
Rhizoma Cimicifugae (*Sheng Ma*)
Radix Angelicae Pubescentis (*Du Huo*)
Radix Angelicae Sinensis (*Dang Gui*)
Radix Et Rhizoma Ligustici Sinensis (*Gao Ben*)
Radix Glycyrrhizae (*Gan Cao*)

Shuang Bai Wan (Double White Pills)

aged Lime (*Shi Hui*), 30g
Sclerotium Poriae Cocos (*Fu Ling*), 60g

Powder and make into pills with water the size of tung seeds. Take 39 pills on an empty stomach. Down with plain, boiled water.

Zhi Dai Wan (Stop Dai Pills)

Radix Angelicae Sinensis (*Dang Gui*)
Radix Ligustici Wallichii (*Chuan Xiong*)
Rhizoma Atractylodis Macrocephalae (*Bai Zhu*)
Radix Panacis Ginseng (*Ren Shen*)

---

[4] This formula was created by Li Dong-yuan. Li's treatment principle of upbearing yang is mentioned numerous times in this chapter by various authors. For more information on meaning and clinical implications of upbearing yang, please see Li Dong-yuan's *Pi Wei Lun (Treatise on the Spleen & Stomach)* translated by Yang Shou-zhong and published by Blue Poppy Press.

Radix Dioscoreae Oppositae (*Shan Yao*)
Cortex Eucommiae Ulmoidis (*Du Zhong*)
Concha Ostreae (*Mu Li*)
Radix Dipsaci (*Xu Duan*)
Fructus Psoraleae Corylifoliae (*Bu Gu Zhi*)
wine stir-fried Cortex Ailanthi Altissimae (*Chu Gen Bai Pi*)
Rhizoma Cyperi Rotundi (*Xiang Fu*)
Pulvis Indigonis (*Qing Dai*)

Make into pills with honey the size of tung seeds. Take on an empty stomach. Drink down with rice soup. Each time take 60 pills. In winter, add mix-fried Radix Glycyrrhizae (*Gan Cao*) and dry Rhizoma Zingiberis (*Gan Jiang*). In summer, add Cortex Phellodendri (*Huang Bai*). If there is abdominal pain which is full and stuffy, delete the Ginseng and add Fructus Amomi (*Sha Ren*).

Shou Dai Liu He Wan (Long-life *Dai* Six Harmonies Pills)

This formula treats red and white *dai xia* and aching and pain in the belly and abdomen. It harmonizes the spleen and stomach, dries dampness in the middle palace, lifts fallen qi, transforms phlegm, and clears fire.

rice-washing water stir-fried Rhizoma Atractylodis Macrocephalae (*Bai Zhu*)
Rhizoma Atractylodis (*Cang Zhu*, prepared as above)
Radix Angelicae Sinensis (*Dang Gui*)
wine stir-fried Radix Albus Paeoniae Lactiflorae (*Bai Shao*)
cooked Radix Rehmanniae (*Shu Di*)
Sclerotium Poriae Cocos (*Fu Ling*), 60g each
Pericarpium Citri Reticulatae (*Chen Pi*)
Radix Glycyrrhizae (*Gan Cao*), 30g each
Rhizoma Pinelliae Ternatae (*Ban Xia*)
wine stir-fried Cortex Ailanthi Altissimae (*Chun Gen Bai Pi*), 45g each
Cortex Radicis Moutan (*Dan Pi*)
Cortex Phellodendri (*Huang Bai*), 36g
Radix Ledebouriellae Divaricatae (*Fang Feng*)
Rhizoma Cimicifugae (*Sheng Ma*), 24g each

Jia Wei Wu Ji San (Added Flavors Five Accumulations Powder)

Treats *dai xia* categorized as vacuity cold. Take *Wu Ji San* (Five Accumulations Powder) plus:

Rhizoma Cyperi Rotundi (*Xiang Fu*)
Fructus Feoniculi Vulgaris (*Xiao Hui Xiang*)
Fructus Corni Officinalis (*Shan Zhu Yu*)

[From Bensky & Barolet's *Chinese Herbal Medicine: Formulas & Strategies*, the standard ingredients of *Wu Ji San*:

Herba Ephedrae (*Ma Huang*), 180g
Radix Angelicae Dahuricae (*Bai Zhi*), 90g
dry Rhizoma Zingiberis (*Gan Jiang*), 120g
Cortex Cinnamomi Cassiae (*Rou Gui*), 90g
Rhizoma Atractylodis (*Cang Zhu*), 720g
Cortex Magnoliae Officinalis (*Hou Po*), 120g
Pericarpium Citri Reticulatae (*Chen Pi*), 180g
Rhizoma Pinelliae Ternatae (*Ban Xia*), 90g
Sclerotium Poriae Cocos (*Fu Ling*), 90g
Radix Platycodi Grandiflori (*Jie Geng*), 360g
Fructus Citri Aurantii (*Zhi Ke*), 180g
Radix Angelicae Sinensis (*Dang Gui*), 90g
Radix Albus Paeoniae Lactiflorae (*Bai Shao*), 90g
Radix Ligustici Wallichii (*Chuan Xiong*), 90g
mix-fried Radix Glycyrrhizae (*Gan Cao*), 90g

Grind into powder. Set aside the Cinnamon and Aurantium. Fry the remaining powder till it changes color and allow it to cool. Add the other two powdered ingredients. Take nine grams as a draft with three slices of uncooked Rhizoma Zingiberis (*Sheng Jiang*).]

Gu Jing Wan (Secure the Essence Pills)

This formula treats *dai xia* categorized as vacuity heat.

Rhizoma Atractylodis Macrocephalae (*Bai Zhu*)
wine stir-fried Radix Albus Paeoniae Lactiflorae (*Bai Shao*), 22.5g each
wine stir-fried Plastrum Testudinis (*Gui Ban*)
wine stir-fried Cortex Phellodendri (*Huang Bai*), 60g each
wine stir-fried Fructus Corni Officinalis (*Shan Zhu Yu*), 15g

Make into pills with rice plaster as big as tung seeds. Take on an empty stomach. Down with clear soup 70-80 pills. If dampness is serious, add 15 grams each of wine stir-fried Cortex Ailanthi Altissimae (*Chun Gen Bai Pi*) and Radix Sophorae Flavescentis (*Ku Shen*) and six grams each of Bulbus Fritillariae (*Bei Mu*) and blast-fried dry Rhizoma Zingiberis (*Pao Gan Jiang*).

Jia Wei Ba Wu Tang (Added Flavors Eight Materials Decoction)

This formula treats *dai xia* categorized as qi and blood vacuity.

Ba Wu (aka *Ba Zhen Tang*) plus:

Radix Dioscoreae Oppositae (*Shan Yao*)
Cortex Eucommiae Ulmoidis (*Du Zhong*)
Rhizoma Cyperi Rotundi (*Xiang Fu*)
uncooked Rhizoma Zingiberis (*Sheng Jiang*)
Fructus Zizyphi Jujubae (*Da Zao*)

Decoct. For fat persons, add Rhizoma Pinelliae Ternatae (*Ban Xia*). For abdominal pain, add Mirabilitum (*Mang Xiao*) and Fructus Feoniculi Vulgaris (*Xiao Hui Xiang*). For abdominal fullness, delete Ginseng. Fennel's nature is dry. It supplements the kidneys and lifegate and treats cold mounting.

[From Bensky & Barolet, the ingredients of *Ba Zhen Tang* are:

Radix Panacis Ginseng (*Ren Shen*)
cooked Radix Rehmanniae (*Shu Di*)
Radix Albus Paeoniae Lactiflorae (*Bai Shao*)
Radix Ligustici Wallichii (*Chuan Xiong*)

Radix Angelicae Sinensis (*Dang Gui*)
Sclerotium Poriae Cocos (*Fu Ling*)
Rhizoma Atractylodis Macrocephalae (*Bai Zhu*)
mix-fried Radix Glycyrrhizae (*Gan Cao*)]

Jia Wei Er Chen Tang (Added Flavors Two Aged [Ingredients] Decoction)

This formula treats *dai xia* categorized as damp heat.

Er Chen plus:

Rhizoma Atractylodis (*Cang Zhu*), 9g
Radix Angelicae Dahuricae (*Bai Zhi*)
Radix Scutellariae Baicalensis (*Huang Qin*), 6g each
Rhizoma Coptidis Chinensis (*Huang Lian*)
Cortex Phellodendri (*Huang Bai*), 4.5g each
Radix Albus Paeoniae Lactiflorae (*Bai Shao*)
Cortex Ailanthi Altissimae (*Chun Gen Bai Pi*)
Fructus Corni Officinalis (*Shan Zhu Yu*), 7.7g each

[From Bensky & Barolet, the ingredients of *Er Chen Tang* are:

Rhizoma Pinelliae Ternatae (*Ban Xia*), 15g
Pericarpium Citri Erythrocarpae (*Ju Hong*), 15g
Sclerotium Poriae Cocos (*Fu Ling*), 9g
mix-fried Radix Glycyrrhizae (*Gan Cao*), 4.5g]

These formulas provide some interesting comparisons with those given in *Nu Ke Mi Jue Da Quan*. Some are the same guiding formula but with varying additions. Different doctors have different styles of prescribing based on differing theories and personal preference. Each variation embodies a potentially different conformation and slightly varying disease mechanism.

Contemporary Chinese Classification & Treatment of *Dai Xia*

Han Bai-ling was a famous Chinese gynecologist who practiced and taught in Harbin, the provincial capital of Heilongjiang in northeast China or what was once known as Manchuria. In *Bai Ling Fu Ke (Bai Ling's Gynecology)*, Dr. Han uses the classical five color categorization for organizing his discussion of *dai xia*.

According to Han Bai-ling, there are two kinds of *dai xia*. The first is physiological *dai xia* and the second is pathological *dai xia*. *Dai xia* like saliva, which is typically moist and a transparent white color, which is neither too much or too little, and has no strange smell is usually physiological, *i.e.*, normal. If the vagina has not been excised and the discharge consists of a turbid white, yellow, greenish, blackish, or red matter with a bad smell, these are species of diseased *dai xia*. Dr. Han quotes from the *Nu Ke Zheng Zhi Yue Ken (Simple & Agreed Upon Treatments for Gynecological Conditions)* when he writes, "If the inside of the vagina has a continuous matter dribbling down drop by drop, this is what is called *dai xia*." He also quotes the *Jin Gui Yao Lue (Essentials from the Golden Cabinet)*: "Thirty-six diseases, namely the three restraints, the five damages, the seven harms, the nine pains, and the 12 lumps."

The Three Restraints: The moon water, *i.e.*, menstruation is dammed and does not flow. There is post partum exhaustion of the breasts, *i.e.*, agalactia. The patient is skinny and emaciated and their flesh is not generated.

The Five Damages: Aperture pain (pain of the vaginal orifice), inside hot and cold pains, irritating, tight pain of the lower abdomen, *ren mai* insensitive or numb, the fetal gate or vagina not straight

The Seven Harms: Food harm, qi harm, chill harm, taxation harm, bedroom harm, *i.e.* sexual harm, pregnancy harm, sleep harm

The Nine Pains: Injury to the inside of the vagina, dribbling pain inside the vagina, pain during urination, cold, chilly pain, abdominal pain at the onset of menstruation, qi replete and concentrated pain, pain and sweating as if gnawed by a worm, bearing down pain from the upper body, lumbar pain

The 12 Lumps: Green mud, green blood, purple juice, red skin, pussy scab, bean juice, plant juice, clotty colored blood, clear blood like water, rice juice, moon wash, amount of menstrual discharge not appropriate for the phase of the flow.

Our ancestors recognized that the above 36 types of women's disease which classically defined gynecology all occur below (*xia*) the *dai (mai)*. Therefore, they were called as a group *dai xia bing* or below the *dai* diseases and gynecologists were called *dai xia yi* or *dai xia* doctors.

The internal causes of *dai xia* as a disease category are stirring of the passions, taxation and servitude beyond measure, immoral sexual intercourse, and an insatiable appetite for uncooked and chilled foods. The external cause is excessive evils which attack the *bao mai* damaging and injuring the *chong* and *ren* which direct the *dai*. Among the most essential factors are damage to both the spleen and kidneys, insufficiency of life fire, loss of spleen warmth, non-transformation of water fluids, and internal accumulation of damp turbidity, all of which may cause loss of restraint of the *dai* and non-securing or non-astringency of the *chong* and *ren*.

In the diagnosis and treatment of *dai xia*, one must be sure to strictly discriminate between hot and cold, vacuity and repletion. Generally, *bai dai* or white *dai* which is clear and thin or watery and smells fishy is categorized as vacuity cold. In that case one should warmly supplement and seep dampness. *Huang dai* or yellow *dai* which is thick and gluey and smells foul is categorized as replete heat. In that case, one should clear heat and drain fire. A yellowish, greenish colored *qing dai* is categorized as damp heat and one should clear heat and disinhibit dampness. Clotty, bloody colored or *hei dai*, black *dai*, is categorized as insufficiency of kidney yang and one ought to boost fire and disperse yin. Red-colored fluid is called *chi dai* and is categorized as vacuity yin/ministerial fire scorching and damaging the *bao mai*. For this, one ought to enrich yin and cool the blood. Red and white *dai xia*, a.k.a. *chi bai dai,* is categorized as damp heat damaging the *bao mai*. For this one ought to clear and disinhibit damp heat. Five-colored *dai, wu se dai,* has a rotten, putrid smell and is categorized as heat toxins damaging and injuring the internal organs. In this case, it is necessary to clear heat, disinhibit dampness, and resolve toxins.

Although the above discussion divides *dai xia* diseases into five types corresponding to the five colors, in present clinical practice, those which commonly present are white *dai*, yellow *dai*, and red and white *dai*. Red *dai*, green *dai*, and black *dai* are usually seen less and five-colored *dai* even less. If it happens that there is a relatively excessive discharge with a foul, unpleasant smell, this suggests a dangerous disease. Excessive desire for sexual intercourse may cause kidney qi to wither and become vacuous. This may result in the discharge of half essence and half blood or the outflow of a gluey, fatty matter called *bai yin* or white looseness. It is also possible for a greyish, whitish colored discharge like rice washing water to be discharged accompanied by inhibition of urination. This is called *bai zhuo* or white turbidity and comes from the bladder. In all kinds of *dai xia* diseases originating within the uterus, one must supplement the kidneys, secure the *chong*, and stop the *dai*. For pathological *dai xia* due to carbuncles and welling abscesses outside the uterus with a thick, bloody discharge, one must clear heat and resolve toxins, quicken the blood and transform stasis. However, in such cases, one must also use surgery and not just rashly fling medicinals to treat this type of *dai*.

Bai Dai

White pathological *dai xia* is mostly caused by excessive fatigue and taxation, undisciplined eating and drinking, non-transformation of the central qi, internal gathering of dampness and turbidity, or insufficiency of kidney yang, lifegate fire not able to warm spleen earth, water dampness eventually damaging the *dai mai*, and lack of astringency of the *chong* and *ren*. Eventually, a white-colored discharge like tears or saliva will flow downward. This is the *bai dai*. As Miao Chong-jing said:

> *Bai dai* mostly is (due to) spleen vacuity and liver qi depression subjugating and (over-)controlling the spleen. When the spleen is damaged, typically damp earth's qi becomes bogged down. Spleen essence is not guarded or kept close and is not able to transform and grow luxuriantly the blood. (Instead, it discharges) downward as a white, slippery matter.

Therefore, *bai dai* is usually categorized as a spleen yang vacuity condition.

Condition's Description: From inside the vagina there is a continuous stream like mucous or saliva which is white in color and fishy smelling. The urination is inhibited, the low back aches, and the body is fatigued. Appetite and thirst are diminished and one's flesh becomes wasted and emaciated. The feces are loose, the face is puffy and the extremities are swollen, and the facial complexion is a somber white. The tongue is pale and wet with white, slimy fur and the pulse is vacuous and slow.

Therapeutic Principles: Fortify the spleen, boost the qi, and seep dampness

Guiding Formula: *Wan Dai Tang* (End *Dai* Decoction) from *Fu Qing Zhu Nu Ke (Fu Qing-zhu's Gynecology)*

Clinical Prescription:

Rhizoma Atractylodis Macrocephalae (*Bai Zhu*), 9g
Radix Dioscoreae Oppositae (*Shan Yao*), 9g
Radix Panacis Ginseng (*Ren Shen*), 12g
Rhizoma Atractylodis (*Cang Zhu*), 9g
Radix Glycyrrhizae (*Gan Cao*), 6g
Pericarpium Citri Reticulatae (*Chen Pi*), 9g
Radix Bupleuri (*Chai Hu*), 6g
Semen Plantaginis (*Che Qian Zi*), 9g
blackened Herba Schizonepetae Tenuifoliae (*Jing Jie*), 6g

In order to fortify the spleen and dry dampness, adding 9 grams of Sclerotium Poriae Cocos (*Fu Ling*) and Semen Euryalis Ferocis (*Qian Shi*) is often beneficial.

Additional Formula: *Wen Shen Zhi Dai Tang* (Warm the Kidneys & Stop *Dai* Decoction) from *Lin Chuang Jing Yan Fang (Empirically Proven Formulas)*

Os Draconis (*Long Gu*), 12g
Concha Ostreae (*Mu Li*), 12g
Radix Dioscoreae Oppositae (*Shan Yao*), 9g
Rhizoma Atractylodis Macrocephalae (*Bai Zhu*), 9g
Sclerotium Poriae Cocos (*Fu Ling*), 12g
Semen Euryalis Ferocis (*Qian Shi*), 12g
Semen Coicis Lachryma-jobi (*Yi Yi Ren*), 12g
Radix Glycyrrhizae (*Gan Cao*), 6g

Huang Dai, Qing Dai

Yellow and greenish *dai* are mostly caused by rash character and excessive anger. The liver does not extend itself and the spleen qi is subjected to (over-)control. The spleen's movement and transformation is then not normal, and dampness and turbidity are not transformed. Depression transforms into heat, and dampness and heat pour downward where they mutually struggle. The *dai mai* fails to restrain and the *chong* and *ren* do not astringe. Thus yellow *dai* is generated. Luo Zhuo-yan said:

> If one has *dai xia* it is because stagnant constructive and defensive qi turn into it. Any cause, such as happiness, anger, worry, or (over-)thinking, post partum or sexual exhaustion, which damage a woman's constructive and defensive, may lead to habitual dampness and heat. This causes a turbid qi to ooze from the bladder which manifests as a mucousy matter which flows downward without stop.

Therefore, yellow and greenish *dai xia* is categorized as a damp heat in the liver channel condition.

Condition's Description: If one has more heat, the discharge will be yellow, thick, gluey, and foul smelling or may be a thick, bloody liquid. The vagina may be burning hot or there may be pain and itching both inside and outside the vagina. Inside the heart, there is irritable and vexatious heat. The mouth is bitter and the throat is dry. There is oral thirst with a desire to drink cold liquids. The stools are constipated and bound and the urination is short and red. The tongue is red with yellow fur, and the pulse is bowstring, slippery, and rapid.

Therapeutic Principles: Clear heat and disinhibit dampness

Guiding Formula: *Long Dan Xie Gan Tang* (Gentiana Drain the Liver Decoction) from *Yi Zong Jin Jian (The Golden Mirror of Ancestral Medicine)*

Clinical Prescription:

Radix Gentianae Scabrae (*Long Dan Cao*), 9g
uncooked Radix Rehmanniae (*Sheng Di*), 9g
Radix Scutellariae Baicalensis (*Huang Qin*), 9g
Fructus Gardeniae Jasminoidis (*Zhi Zi*), 9g
Caulis Akebiae (*Mu Tong*), 6g
Semen Plantaginis (*Che Qian Zi*), 9g
Rhizoma Alismatis (*Ze Xie*), 9g
Radix Angelicae Sinensis (*Dang Gui*), 6g
Radix Bupleuri (*Chai Hu*), 6g
Radix Glycyrrhizae (*Gan Cao*), 6g

If one has scanty urine, add a small amount of Radix Et Rhizoma Rhei (*Da Huang*). If there is hemafecia, add 9 grams of Cortex Ailanthi Altissimae (*Chen Gen Bai Pi*) and Herba Et Radix Cirsii Japonici (*Xiao Ji*). If the stools are loose and the vagina is swollen, add 12 grams of Herba Artemisiae Capillaris (*Yin Chen Hao*) and 9 grams of Sclerotium Rubrum Poriae Cocos (*Chi Fu Ling*).

External Medicinals [for the treatment of swelling and pain of the inside and outside of the vagina with possible ulceration and erosion]

Medicinal Wash:

Radix Sophorae Flavescentis (*Ku Shen*), 15g
Fructus Cnidii Monnieri (*She Chuang Zi*), 15g
Fructus Carpesii Abrotanoidis (*Hei Shi*), 15g
Radix Stemonae (*Bai Bu*), 15g
Cortex Phellodendri (*Huang Bai*), 9g
Alumen (*Ku Fan*), 6g
Realgar (*Xiong Huang*), 9g

Decoct in water and strain out the dregs, fumigate and wash the affected part.

Medicinals for Direct Application:

Alumen (*Ku Fan*), 6g
Acacia Catechu (*Er Cha*), 6g
Realgar (*Xiong Huang*), 9g
Os Draconis (*Long Gu*), 9g
Borneolum (*Bing Pian*), 3g
Cortex Phellodendri (*Huang Bai*), 6g

Grind the above medicinals into a fine powder and gently, gently apply to the affected area. This formula is capable of killing germs, stopping itching, and engendering new tissue.

Chi Bai Dai

Red and white *dai xia* is mostly caused by damp heat within the body or vacuity of the sea of blood either at the time of menstruation or post partum. Externally, one may be subjected to rain, fog, and dew, *i.e.*, external dampness, or one may have an addiction to uncooked, chilled foods. Inside the body, yang qi is depressed and shut and cold dampness invades and assails the *bao mai*. This causes damage and injury to the *chong* and *ren* which results in lack of restraint of the *dai mai*. Therefore, this condition is categorized as cold damp damage and injury to the *bao mai*.

Condition's Description: There is red and white *dai xia*. Either red or white colored discharge may preponderate. The menstruation is excessive and is interlocked behind (the damp heat. This may also imply the menses is behind schedule). There is cold pain with urination and the vagina inside feels heavy and distended. There is low back pain and the body feels weary, the four extremities may change abruptly from cold to hot, and the facial color is dull and stagnant. The tongue is pale and wet with white, slimy fur. The pulse is bowstring and moderate (*i.e.*, relaxed or slightly slow).

Therapeutic Principles: Warm the menses, disinhibit dampness, and stop bleeding and *dai xia*

Guiding Formula: *Yu Ai Si Wu Zhi Dai Tang* (Sanguisorba & Mugwort Four Materials Stop *Dai* Decoction) from *Lin Chuang Jing Yan Fang (Empirically Proven Formulas)*

Clinical Prescription:

Radix Angelicae Sinensis (*Dang Gui*), 9g
Radix Ligustici Wallichii (*Chuan Xiong*), 6g
Radix Albus Paeoniae Lactiflorae (*Bai Shao*), 12g
cooked Radix Rehmanniae (*Shu Di*), 9g
Folium Artemisiae Argyii (*Ai Ye*), 9g
Radix Achyranthis Bidentatae (*Niu Xi*), 9g
Rhizoma Atractylodis (*Cang Zhu*), 9g
Sclerotium Poriae Cocos (*Fu Ling*), 9g
Radix Polygalae Tenuifoliae (*Yuan Zhi*), 6g
Radix Glycyrrhizae (*Gan Cao*), 6g
stir-fried Radix Sanguisorbae (*Di Yu*), 15g

If there is mostly red discharge and the vagina is burning hot, delete the Artemesia Argyium and add nine grams or Radix Scutellariae Baicalensis (*Huang Qin*) and Cortex Ailanthi Altissimae (*Chun Gen Bai Pi*) in order to clear heat and stop bleeding.

Clotty Colored *Hei Dai*

Hei dai or black *dai* is mostly caused by kidney qi depletion and decline and lifegate fire insufficiency or excessive venal desire for sexual intercourse. Yin essence may thus be consumed and fat and grease are not engendered. Damp turbidity damages and injures the *dai mai,* and the *chong* and *ren* fail to astringe. According to the *Fu Ren Da Quan Liang Fang (The Great Compendium of Fine Formulas for Women)*:

> Women's *dai xia* is of five different types. It is caused by menstruation going (the wrong way) after delivery. Wind evils enter the gate to the uterus and are thence transmitted to the viscera and bowels. This results in ... damage to the foot *shao yin* kidney channel. A black, clotted, blood-colored discharge and violent pain across the waist as if bound tightly by a belt arises from this and, for that reason, this disease is called *dai,* belt.

This condition is categorized as a species of kidney qi depletion and decline.

Condition's Description: There is a dirty, turbid discharge like clotty blood which is continuous and does not stop. The low back aches and the legs are weak. The abdomen is chilly and the extremities are cold. There is polyuria and loose stools. The four extremities are not warm, the head is dizzy and forgetful, and the facial color is gloomy and dull. The tongue is pale and wet and the pulse is deep and weak.

Therapeutic Principles: Enrich the kidneys, fortify the spleen, and eliminate dampness

Guiding Formula: *Jia Wei Bu Shen Gu Jing Wan* (Added Flavors Supplement the Kidneys & Secure the Essence Pills) from *Lin Chuang Jing Yan Fang (Empirically Proven Formulas)*

Clinical Prescription:

Radix Panacis Ginseng (*Ren Shen*), 9g
Rhizoma Atractylodis Macrocephalae (*Bai Zhu*), 9g

Cortex Eucommiae Ulmoidis (*Du Zhong*), 9g
Radix Dipsaci (*Xu Duan*), 9g
Semen Coicis Lachryma-jobi (*Yi Yi Ren*), 9g
Gelatinum Corii Asini (*E Jiao*), 9g
Folium Artemisiae Argyii (*Ai Ye*), 9g
Semen Cuscutae Chinensis (*Tu Si Zi*), 9g
Fructus Psoraleae Corylifoliae (*Bu Gu Zhi*), 9g

To this add:

Radix Dioscoreae Oppositae (*Shan Yao*), 9g
Os Draconis (*Long Gu*), 12g
Hallyositum Rubrum (*Chi Shi Zhi*), 12g

Chi Dai

If the *dai xia* is red and liquidy like water with a hot and painful urinary tract and there is lumbar pain when one rolls over, the heart is vexed and not calm, and there is heat in the center of the hands and feet, tidal fever and night sweats, a red face with malar flushing, a red tongue with no fur, a dry mouth with no saliva, and a bowstring, fine, and rapid pulse, this is categorized as kidney yin vacuity *dai xia*.

Therapeutic Principles: Enrich yin, supplement the kidneys, and cool the blood

Guiding Formula: *Yang Yin Liang Xue Zhi Dai Tang* (Nourish Yin, Cool the Blood & Stop *Dai* Decoction) from *Lin Chuang Jing Yan Fang (Empirically Proven Formulas)*

Clinical Prescription:

uncooked Radix Rehmanniae (*Sheng Di*), 9g
Radix Achyranthis Bidentatae (*Niu Xi*), 9g
Cortex Ailanthi Altissimae (*Chun Gen Bai Pi*), 9g
Cortex Radicis Moutan (*Dan Pi*), 9g
Radix Albus Paeoniae Lactiflorae (*Bai Shao*), 12g

stir-fried Radix Sanguisorbae (*Di Yu*), 12g
Gelatinum Corii Asini (*E Jiao*), 9g
Tuber Ophiopogonis Japonici (*Mai Dong*), 9g
Fructus Lycii Chinensis (*Gou Qi Zi*), 6g
Cortex Phellodendri (*Huang Bai*), 6g

Wu Se Dai

Five-colored *dai* is mostly due to habitual visceral vacuity, enduring combination of dampness and heat, and heat toxins damaging and injuring the *bao mai*. Therefore, this condition is categorized as damp toxin damage and injury of the internal viscera.

Condition's Description: There is five-colored vaginal discharge with a foul, unpleasant smell. Inside the vagina there is a burning pain which feels weighed down and distended. The heart is anxious and not calm, the mouth is thirsty and the throat is dry, the feces are either withheld or loose and unformed, the urine is red, there is heat in the center of the hands and feet, and the facial color lacks luster. The tongue fur is sticky and slimy, and the pulse is bowstring, slippery, and moderate (*i.e.,* relaxed or slightly slow).

Therapeutic Principles: Clear heat, resolve toxins, and transform dampness

Guiding Formula: *Jie Du Zhi Dai Tang* (Resolve Toxins & Stop *Dai* Decoction) from *Lin Chuang Jing Yan Fang (Empirically Proven Formulas)*

Clinical Prescription:

Flos Lonicerae Japonicae (*Jin Yin Hua*), 12g
Fructus Forsythiae Suspensae (*Lian Qiao*), 9g
Radix Sophorae Flavescentis (*Ku Shen*), 9g
Herba Artemisiae Capillaris (*Yin Chen Hao*), 12g
Cortex Phellodendri (*Huang Bai*), 6g
Radix Scutellariae Baicalensis (*Huang Qin*), 9g

Radix Albus Paeoniae Lactiflorae (*Bai Shao*), 12g
Cortex Ailanthi Altissimae (*Chun Gen Bai Pi*), 9g
Radix Achyranthis Bidentatae (*Niu Xi*), 9g
uncooked Radix Rehmanniae (*Sheng Di*), 9g
Cortex Radicis Moutan (*Dan Pi*), 9g
Rhizoma Guanchong (*Guan Zhong*), 9g
Rhizoma Coptidis Chinensis (*Huang Lian*), 9g
stir-fried Radix Sanguisorbae (*Di Yu*), 12g

External Medicinals [for the treatment of swelling and pain inside and outside the vagina with possible ulceration and erosion]

Medicinal Wash

Radix Sophorae Flavescentis (*Ku Shen*), 15g
Fructus Cnidii Monnieri (*She Chuang Zi*), 15g
Fructus Carpesii Abrotanoidis (*Hei Shi*), 15g
Radix Stemonae (*Bai Bu*), 15g
Cortex Phellodendri (*Huang Bai*), 9g
Alumen (*Ku Fan*), 6g
Realgar (*Xiong Huang*), 9g

Decoct in water and strain out the dregs. Fumigate and wash the affected area.

Medicinals for Direct Application:

Alumen (*Ku Fan*), 6g
Acacia Catechu (*Er Cha*), 6g
Realgar (*Xiong Huang*), 9g
Os Draconis (*Long Gu*), 9g
Borneolum (*Bing Pian*), 3g
Cortex Phellodendri (*Huang Bai*), 6g

Grind into a fine powder and carefully apply to the affected area. This prescription is capable of killing germs, stopping itching, and engendering new tissue.

More modern TCM gynecology clinical manuals, such as *Fu Ke Zheng Zhi (Gynecological Patterns & Treatments)* published in Hebei in 1983, typically merely say that *dai xia* is due to insufficiency of kidney qi, lack of strength of spleen movement, *ren mai* not astringing or securing, *dai mai* not restraining, and the possibility of disease evils causing internal damage.

Sun Jiu-ling, the author of *Fu Ke Zheng Zhi*, discriminates only three basic categories of *dai xia*: spleen vacuity, kidney vacuity, and damp toxins.

Spleen Vacuity

Sun Jiu-ling gives the signs and symptoms of this pattern as a continuous white discharge, possibly yellowish but without offensive odor, a sallow, yellowish facial complexion, lack of warmth in the four extremities, listlessness of the essence spirit, fatigue, lack of strength, loose, thin, flimsy stools, slightly swollen lower extremities, a pale tongue with white, possibly sticky, slimy fur, and a moderate (*i.e.*, relaxed, slightly slow), weak pulse.

Because the spleen is vacuous and weak, it is incapable of moving and transforming water dampness. Water dampness therefore pours downward causing *dai xia*. Spleen vacuity and, hence, lack of forceful upbearing of central yang result in the facial complexion not being nourished and thus sallow yellow, the four extremities lacking warmth, and the demeanor being weary and tired. The spleen's lacking the strength for movement results in the stools' being loose, the lower extremities' being slightly swollen, the tongue pale with white or slimy fur, and the pulse moderate and weak.

Sun lists the therapeutic principles for treating this pattern of *dai xia* as fortifying the spleen and boosting the qi, upbearing yang, and eliminating dampness. For these purposes, Sun recommends *Wan Dai Tang* discussed above. Sun then goes on to say that dampness may transform into heat, thus creating a damp hot condition. In this case, the *dai* will be yellow in color, gluey, and thick with offensive odor. In this case, the therapeutic principles are to clear heat, disinhibit dampness, and stop *dai* for which Sun suggests *Yi Huang Tang*. A similar formula with the same name has been described above. However, since Sun's version is different, it is given below

Radix Dioscoreae Oppositae (*Shan Yao*), 30g
Semen Euryalis Ferocis (*Qian Shi*), 15g
Semen Plantaginis (*Che Qian Zi*), 30g
Semen Gingkonis Bilobae (*Bai Guo*), 6g
Cortex Phellodendri (*Huang Bai*), 9g
Rhizoma Alismatis (*Ze Xie*), 9g
Caulis Akebiae (*Mu Tong*), 9g

Decoct in water two times and divide the resulting liquid into three portions. Take one portion three times per day.

Kidney Vacuity

Sun Jiu-ling gives the signs and symptoms of this pattern as a clear white, chilly discharge, excessive in amount and thin in consistency. There is lumbar soreness and pain and the knees lack strength. The urine is clear and copious and the stools are loose, thin, and flimsy. The tongue is pale with thin, white fur, and the pulse is deep and fine.

Because kidney yang is insufficient, yin cold accumulates internally and the *dai mai* cannot restrain. The *ren mai* fails to secure and astringe and thus the *dai xia* is clear and chilly, is excessive in amount, and is thin in consistency. Because kidney yang is insufficient, lifegate fire wanes and is unable to warm the bladder below. This results in the urination being frequent, clear, and long. Above, it is incapable of warming spleen yang and this results in the stools being loose, thin, and flimsy below. The low back is the mansion of the kidneys and kidney vacuity results in low back soreness and pain and the knees' lacking strength. The uterus is located in the lower abdomen and the *bao mai* homes to the kidneys. Kidney yang vacuity and waning is incapable of warming the uterus and thus the lower abdomen feels chilly. The tongue is pale with thin, white fur and the pulse

Dai Xia/Abnormal Vaginal Discharge

is deep and fine because kidney yang is insufficient to go on a journey upward.

Sun gives the therapeutic principles for treating this pattern of *dai xia* as warming the kidneys and invigorating yang, securing, astringing, and stopping *dai*. For this purpose, Sun recommends *Fu Fang Ba Wei Wan Jia Jian* (Compound Eight Flavors Pills with Additions & Subtractions).

cooked Radix Rehmanniae (*Shu Di*), 30g
Rhizoma Alismatis (*Ze Xie*), 9g
Sclerotium Poriae Cocos (*Fu Ling*), 15g
Fructus Corni Officinalis (*Shan Zhu Yu*), 9g
Radix Dioscoreae Oppositae (*Shan Yao*), 15g
Radix Lateralis Praeparatus Aconiti Carmichaeli (*Fu Zi*), 9g
Cortex Cinnamomi Cassiae (*Rou Gui*), 9g
Fructus Foeniculi Vulgaris (*Xiao Hui Xiang*), 9g
Fructus Psoraleae Corylifoliae (*Bu Gu Zhi*), 9g
Flos Celosiae Cristatae (*Ji Guan Hua*), 15g

Decoct in water two times, divide the resulting liquid into three portions, and take one portion three times per day.

Damp Toxins

Sun Jiu-ling gives the signs and symptoms of this pattern as excessive vaginal discharge which is yellow or green in color and thick, possibly mixed with a bloody liquid, possibly with a fishy stench or like rice-washing water, vaginal ulceration and itching, short, reddish urination, a bitter taste in the mouth and dry throat, a red tongue with yellow fur, and a slippery, rapid pulse.

Damp toxins invade internally. This accumulation generates heat which damages and injures the *chong* and *ren mai*. Dirty turbidity flows downward and causes *dai xia* like rice-washing water, thick, yellowish green, or mixed with bloody liquid with an offensive stench and itching and ulceration of the vagina. Damp heat accumulating internally damages the fluids and humor sand causes a bitter taste in the mouth, dryness of

Fire In The Valley

the throat, and scanty, red urine. The red tongue with yellow fur and the rapid pulse are due to damp toxins invading internally and transforming into heat.

Sun lists the therapeutic principles for treating this pattern as clearing heat and resolving toxins, disinhibiting dampness and stopping *dai*. For these purposes, Sun suggests *Jia Wei Dai Xia Tang* (Added Flavors *Dai Xia* Decoction).

Rhizoma Smilacis Glabrae (*Tu Fu Ling*), 30g
Flos Lonicerae Japonicae (*Jin Yin Hua*), 15g
Pericarpium Citri Reticulatae (*Chen Pi*), 9g
Radix Gentianae Scabrae (*Long Dan Cao*), 9g
Fructus Gardeniae Jasminoidis (*Zhi Zi*), 9g
Caulis Akebiae (*Mu Tong*), 9g
Radix Et Rhizoma Rhei (*Da Huang*), 9g
Sclerotium Poriae Cocos (*Fu Ling*), 15g
Radix Achyranthis Bidentatae (*Niu Xi*), 12g

Decoct in water two times, divide into three portions, and take one portion three times per day.

Zhu Cheng-han, author of *Zhong Yi Fu Ke (Chinese Gynecology)* gives a different but equally useful formula for the treatment of *dai xia* due to damp toxins in the *bao gong*. The formula is called *Qing Gong Li Dai Tang* (Clear the Uterus & Disinhibit *Dai* Decoction) and is for the purpose of clearing heat and resolving toxins. It is composed of:

Herba Violae Yedoensitis Cum Radice (*Zi Hua Di Ding*), 30g
Herba Taraxaci Mongolici Cum Radice (*Pu Gong Ying*), 30g
Radix Scutellariae Baicalensis (*Huang Qin*), 9g
Cortex Phellodendri (*Huang Bai*), 9g
Herba Patriniae Heterophyllae Cum Radice (*Bai Jiang Cao*), 9g
Radix Sophorae Flavescentis (*Ku Shen*), 9g
Cortex Ailanthi Altissimae (*Chun Gen Bai Pi*), 12g
Semen Plantaginis (*Che Qian Zi*), 9g
Radix Albus Paeoniae Lactiflorae (*Bai Shao*), 9g

Radix Rubrus Paeoniae Lactiflorae (*Chi Shao*), 9g
Radix Glycyrrhizae (*Gan Cao*), 4.5g

The Acupuncture Treatment of *Dai Xia*

Cheng Dan-An

Prior to the rise of TCM as a modern style with its emphasis on treatment based on the discrimination of patterns, most clinical Chinese acupuncture literature was arranged according to *bian bing lun zhi* or treatment based on the discrimination of diseases. Cheng Dan-an's discussion of the acupuncture treatment of *dai xia* is representative of this pre-TCM acupuncture literature. Cheng Dan-an was a famous early 20th Century acupuncturist practicing in Nanjing and Zhejiang province.

In *Cheng Dan An Zhen Jiu Xuan Ji (The Selected Acupuncture Writings of Cheng Dan-an)*, Cheng begins with a discussion of the disease causes of *dai xia*: Evil heat is a guest in the uterus and causes *dai xia*. If it becomes mingled with blood there is red *dai* and is due to heat. Faint urination gives rise to pain and the vagina is burning hot. The matter discharged from the place below may be mingled with filth and may smell. The cold type is not painful and has no filthy, foul smell. The matter discharged from the place below is white-colored and excessive. This may also be caused by excessive worry and thought, hand looseness, *i.e.*, masturbation, and immorality in bedroom affairs.

Cheng gives the signs and symptoms of *dai xia* as excessive discharge similar to water or like pus. If it is white in color it is called *bai dai*, and if it is red in color it is called *chi dai*. The uterus may ache and the urination may be frequent, incomplete, and so smelly as to be unendurable. If this condition is not treated properly, this pasty, gluey fluid will increase.

Treatment:
Needle *Gui Lai* (St 29)
    "   *Zhong Ji* (CV 3)
    "   *San Yin Jiao* (Sp 6), also moxa 5 cones
    "   *Xue Hai* (Sp 10)
Moxa *Shen Shu* (Bl 23) and *Guan Yuan* (CV 4) 5-7 cones each

Adjunctive Therapy: Decoct 15 grams of the heart of sunflower stem with several pieces of Fructus Zizyphi Jujubae (*Da Zao*) and a suitable amount of brown sugar and take.

Prognosis: Mostly good. If one has a complicated condition there is no certainty of cure.

Tian Cong-huo

This methodology for discussing the acupuncture-moxibustion treatment of *dai xia* is still current today as witnessed by Tian Cong-huo's discussion in *Zhen Jiu Yi Xue Yan Ji (A Collection of Tested Acupuncture-moxibustion Medical Theories)*. Tian Cong-huo discusses *dai xia* under the rubric of *bai dai* or leukorrhea which is a common practice in the Chinese medical literature.[5] Tian says that leukorrhea describes vaginal secretions which are excessive in quantity and white in color which usually arise together with or are interconnected with some inflammatory condition, tumors, constitutional vacuity weakness, or other such causes. This what is traditionally called *dai xia*. It mostly has to do with damp heat pouring downward or qi and blood vacuity detriment. In clinical practice, most white colored *dai xia* is due to physiological causes. A white-colored discharge which is milky and pasty in appearance is mostly due to vaginitis associated with hemophilus. A pussy discharge is mostly due to trichomoniasis or possibly to atrophic vaginitis. If there is foreign

---

[5] In other words, now in Chinese medicine, *bai dai* may mean either a specifically white *dai* or it may mean leukorrhea and be used a generic term for all abnormal vaginal discharges.

matter inside the vagina which is like a gluey liquid, this is mostly due to chronic cervicitis or cervical polyps. If there is a watery, bloody discharge which is foul smelling, such *bai dai* is mostly due to tumor.

Fine Needle Treatment

Selected Points For Use

Main Points: *Dai Mai* (GB 26), *San Yin Jiao* (Sp 6), & *Qi Hai* (CV 6)

Auxiliary Points: *Guan Yuan* (CV 4), *Zu San Li* (St 36), *Yin Ling Quan* (Sp 9), *Nei Guan* (Per 6), *Shen Men* (Ht 7), *Jian Shi* (Per 5), *Shen Shu* (Bl 23), *Zhi Shi* (Bl 52), *Ming Men* (GV 4), & *Xing Jian* (Liv 2)

Empirically Proven Points: *Huan Tiao* (GB 30) & *Si Hua Xue* (the four flowers points, *i.e.*, *Ge Shu* [Bl 17] & *Dan Shu* [Bl 19])

Needle Stimulation Method: Commonly one uses the even supplementing/even draining or supplementation methods for the main or ruling points. It is possible to also add moxibustion. In repletion patterns, it is okay to use draining method. Retain the needles for 15-20 minutes. Treat one time per day with 10 treatments equaling one course of therapy.

Empirically Proven Experience:

Twenty-eight persons were treated for *bai dai* with acupuncture-moxibustion. The main points were the *Si Hua Xue*. If the menses were irregular, *Nei Guan* and *San Yin Jiao* were also used. If there were heart palpitations, *Nei Guan* and *Shen Men* were added. If there was low back pain and lack of strength of the four extremities, *Shen Shu, Dai Mai, Zu San Li,* and *Yin Ling Quan* were also used. If there was yellowish red *dai xia* signifying heat, needle stimulation was draining. For heart palpitations, lumbar pain, and malaise, supplementation was used or warming moxibustion added. Of the 28 patients treated thus, 21 experienced complete relief, six improved, and only one experienced no improvement. Typically, these patients got better with only 3-4 treatments. Most recovered with only six treatments.

Tian Cong-huo's discussion of the acupuncture-moxibustion treatment of *dai xia* adds further differential diagnosis and adjustment of the guiding formula based on pattern discrimination. In addition, in Tian's discussion, Western medical etiologies take the place of classical Chinese disease causes and disease mechanisms. This same methodology of advancing a basic acupuncture formula for treating the disease category *dai xia* which can then be modified by the addition of various subsidiary points based on *bian zheng lun zhi* is also used by Zhu Cheng-han in *Zhong Yi Fu Ke (Chinese Medicine Gynecology)*. However, Zhu uses somewhat different points.

Main Points: *Guan Yuan* (CV 4) & *Di Ji* (Sp 8)

Auxiliary Points: If there is spleen vacuity, add *San Yin Jiao* (Sp 6) and *Pi Shu* (Bl 20). If there is kidney vacuity, add *Shen Shu* (Bl 23) and *Tai Xi* (Ki 3). If here is damp heat, add *Yin Ling Quan* (Sp 9) and *Xing Jian* (Liv 2) and replace *Guan Yuan* with *Zhong Ji* (CV 3).

In addition, Zhu also gives an ear needling therapy: Ear Uterus, Ovary, Inside Heart Secret, Liver, Spleen, Kidneys, and other such points.

Xiao Shao-qing

The movement within TCM to herbalize the methodology of acupuncture based on *bian zheng lun zhi* or the formulation of treatment based on a discrimination of patterns reaches its apogee in Xiao Shao-qing's *Zhong Yi Zhen Jiu Chu Fang Xue (A Study of Writing Chinese Medicine Acupuncture-Moxibustion Prescriptions)*. Xiao Shao-qing is a professor of acupuncture-moxibustion at the Nanjing College of Chinese Medicine. His book approaches the practice of acupuncture as if one were writing a TCM herbal prescription.

Xiao divides his discussion of the acupuncture-moxibustion treatment of *dai xia (bai dai)* according to TCM therapeutic principles. Xia then gives a guiding formula, the *bian zheng* indications for this formula, and a number of modifications with auxiliary points for idiosyncracies in presenting symptoms. Xiao then gives a theoretical rationalization for the points used and ends with a selection of classical cites supporting each points empirical usage.

1. Clearing Heat, Disinhibiting Dampness, Stopping *Dai* Formula

Guiding Formula: *Dai Mai* (GB 26), *Bai Huan Shu* (Bl 30), *Qi Hai* (CV 6), *Xing Jian* (Liv 2), & *Yin Ling Quan* (Sp 9)

Indications: *Dai xia* (damp heat type): *Dai xia* of recent onset, a sticky, viscous, yellow colored discharge with a foul smell, dry stool, short, reddish urine, pulse soft and fast, tongue fur yellow and slimy. The *dai* may also be colored simultaneously red, the mouth may have a bitter taste, the throat may be dry, and the five centers may experience vexatious heat. There may be heart palpitations, loss of sleep, impatient mood, rashness, and easy irritation, and the pulse may be soft, bowstring, and rapid with yellow tongue fur.

Additional Points Depending Upon the Presenting Condition:

If there are heart palpitations and insomnia, add *Shen Men* (Ht 7) & *Tai Xi* (Ki 3).

If the stools are dry, add *Tian Shu* (St 25) & *Da Dun* (Liv 1).

Formula Rationalization: *Dai Mai* is chosen to astringe and secure the channel qi and therefore treat pathological discharge. *Bai Huan Shu* and *Qi Hai* are able to promote the free flow and balance the *ren mai* and help the bladder qi to transform evil dampness. *Xing Jian* is chosen to drain evil heat from the liver channel. *Yin Ling Quan* is used to clear and eliminate damp heat from the spleen channel. When these points are used together, their effect is to clear heat, eliminate dampness, and stop *dai*.

Verification of the Functions of These Points:

1. *Dai Mai*: The *Zhen Jiu Da Cheng (Great Compendium of Acupuncture-moxibustion)* says: "Treats irregular menstruation, red and white *dai xia*." The *Zhen Jiu Xue (The Study of Acupuncture-moxibustion)* says: "Treats menstrual irregularity, *dai xia*."

2. *Bai Huan Shu*: The *Lie Jing Tu Yi (The Illustrated Appendix to the Systematized Classic)* says: "For the treatment of dream loss white turbidity, kidney vacuity lumbar pain, first drain, then supplement; red *dai*, drain; menstrual irregularity, also supplement."

3. *Qi Hai*: The *Zhong Hua Zhen Jiu Xue (The Study of Chinese Acupuncture-moxibustion)* says: "Treats red and white *dai xia*, irregular menstruation."

4. *Xing Jian*: The *Lei Jing Tu Yi (The Illustrated Appendix to the Systematized Classic)* says: "Treats red urine, difficulty urinating, white turbidity, distention and pain of the chest, upper back, heart, and abdomen. Draining *Xing Jian* automatically clears fire and heat and wood qi is automatically descended."

5. *Yin Ling Quan*: The *Zhen Jiu Xue (The Study of Acupuncture-moxibustion)* says: "*Yin Ling Quan* is capable of transforming damp *dai*, disinhibiting the lower burner."

2. Boosting the Middle, Fortifying the Spleen, Seeping Dampness Formula

Guiding Formula: *Guan Yuan* (CV 4), *Dai Mai* (GB 26), *Zu San Li* (St 36), & *San Yin Jiao* (Sp 6)

Indications: *Dai xia* (cold damp type): Chronic *dai xia*, watery, thin discharge white in color with a raw odor but no foul smell. There is a heavy, aching pain in the low back, the head is dizzy, and there is a lack of spirit. The extremities and the body are tired and exhausted. The appetite is poor, the stools are loose, and the extremities are chilled. The pulse is soft, slow, bowstring or deep and moderate (*i.e.* relaxed or slightly slow). The tongue fur is thin, white, and slimy.

Additional Points Depending Upon the Presenting Condition:

If there is lack of appetite, add *Zhong Wan* (CV 12), *Zhang Men* (Liv 13), & *Pi Shu* (Bl 20).

If the stools are loose or there is diarrhea, add *Tian Shu* (St 25) & *Da Chang Shu* (Bl 25).

Formula Rationalization: The root formula possesses the ability to boost the middle, disperse cold, fortify the spleen, seep dampness, and balance and supplement the *ren* and *dai mai*. *Guan Yuan* and *Zu San Li* can disinhibit and secure the lower source and can fortify the spleen and seep dampness. *Dai Mai Xue* is capable of astringing the channel qi and regulating *dai* diseases. *San Yin Jiao* and *Zu San Li* used together have the power to fortify the spleen and seep dampness and balance and supplement the liver and kidneys.

Verification of the Functions of These Points:

1. *Guan Yuan*: The *Lei Jing Tu Yi (The Illustrated Appendix to the Systematized Classic)* says: "Treats all the hundreds of vacuity diseases, white turbidity, the five stranguries, women's *dai xia*, abdominal lumps, and lack of free flow of the menstruate."

2. *Dai Mai*: The *Zhong Guo Zhen Jiu Xue (The Study of Chinese Acupuncture-moxibustion)* says: "Treats irregular menstruation, red and white *dai xia*."

3. *Zu San Li*: The *Zhen Jiu Xue Jian Bian (A Concise Study of Acupuncture-moxibustion)* says: "Treats a very wide group of patterns; especially used for digestive system diseases. Also good for diseases of the circulatory, respiratory, and genitourinary systems. This is the single

most important point for the health of the entire body. Treats ... *dai xia*, vomiting in pregnancy, post partum abdominal pain..."

4. *San Yin Jiao*: The *Zhen Jiu Xue Jian Bian (A Concise Study of Acupuncture-moxibustion)* says: "This frequently used, effective point treats diseases of the digestive system and the genitourinary system. Treats spleen-stomach vacuity weakness, jammed full distention of the heart and abdomen, lack of desire for food and drink, abdominal distention with intestinal noises, diarrhea, indigestion; used in women's abdominal lumps, flooding and leaking, menstrual irregularity, painful menstruation, blocked menstruation (or amenorrhea), *dai xia*..."

Added References

1. In this disease, the vagina continuously oozes and discharges various kinds of pasty, greasy, fluidy matter. White and yellow *dai* are the two most commonly met varieties. White *dai* is seen twice as often as red *dai*. The pattern discrimination of this condition is divided into two types: damp heat and cold dampness.

2. The root of this disease is a discharge condition which is due to the *ren mai* not astringing and loss of restraint of the *dai mai* so that water, dampness, turbidity, and fluids pour down and accumulate. It is also possible that intemperate food and drink damage the spleen and stomach which then let slip their job of movement and transformation. Thus damp qi is not moved and turns into *dai xia*. Yellow *dai* is mostly caused by spleen heat. White *dai* is mostly caused by vacuity cold. If one's aspirations do not unfold as desired, liver qi may become stagnant and bound. Enduring evils transform into heat and this heat and blood wrestle together. Damp heat pours downward, and this typically turns into red *dai* or red and white *dai*.

3. Present day medical theory: *Dai xia* refers to an increased amount of vaginal excreta than is normal during a given period of time. It typically accompanies infection in the reproductive organs, such as vaginitis, cervicitis, pelvic inflammatory disease, etc. It may also be related to tumors and constitutional emptiness and weakness.

Dai Xia/Abnormal Vaginal Discharge

4. The method of treating this disease: Choose *ren mai, dai mai*, and foot three yin channel points to treat this. For damp heat, needle with draining technique and do not use moxa. For cold dampness, needle with even supplementing/even draining technique and use lots of moxa. Retain the needles 20 minutes. Treat one time per day; 10 treatments equal one course.

Selected Recorded Effective Formulas:

1. *Guan Yuan* (CV 4) treats *dai xia* and abdominal lumps. *Qi Hai* (CV 6) and *Xiao Chang Shu* (Bl 27) treat *dai*. *Zhong Ji* (CV 3) treats *dai xia*, irregular menstruation. *Dai Mai* (GB 26) treats red and white *dai xia*. *San Yin Jiao* (Sp 6) treats *da xia*. And *Qu Gu* (CV 2) treats red and white *dai xia*. (*Zhen Jiu Zi Sheng Jing [The Acupuncture-moxibustion Classic for Nourishing Life]*)

2. Red and white *dai xia*: *Dai Mai* (GB 26), *Guan Yuan* (CV 4), *Qi Hai* (CV 6), *San Yin Jiao* (Sp 6), *Ba Huan Shu* (Bl 30), & *Jian Shi* (Per 5). (*Shen Ying Jing [The Divinely Responding Classic]*)

3. Drenching *dai*, red and white: *Ming Men* (GV 4), *Shen Que* (CV 8), & *Zhong Ji* (CV 3), moxa each 7 cones. (*Lei Jing Tu Yi [The Illustrated Appendix to the Systematized Classic]; Zhen Jiu Yao Lan [Essential Readings in Acupuncture-moxibustion]*)

4. Red and white *dai xia*: *Qi Hai* (CV 6), *Zhong Ji* (CV 3), *Bai Huan Shu* (Bl 30), *Shen Shu* (Bl 23), *San Yin Jiao* (Sp 6), & *Yang Jiao* (GB 35). (*Zhen Jiu Da Cheng [The Great Compendium of Acupuncture-moxibustion]*) (However, in my copy of Yang Ji-zhou's *Zhen Jiu Da Cheng*, in the gynecology section under red and white *dai xia*, it says: *Dai Mai* (GB 26), *Guan Yuan* (CV 4), *San Yin Jiao* (Sp 6), *Bai Huan Shu* (Bl 30), and *Jian Shi* (Per 5) [30 cones].)

5. *Bai dai*: *Dai Mai* (GB 26), *Zhong Ji* (CV 3), *Shen Shu* (Bl 23), *Gan Shu* (Bl 18), *Pi Shu* (Bl 20), & *San Yin Jiao* (Sp 6), moxa each 3-5 cones. (*Zhong Hua Zhen Jiu Xue [The Study of Chinese Acupuncture-moxibustion]*)

6. Red *dai*: *Dai Mai* (GB 26), *Gan Shu* (Bl 18), *Pi Shu* (Bl 20), *San Yin Jiao* (Sp 6), *Qi Hai* (CV 6), *Zhong Ji* (CV 3), *Xue Hai* (Sp 10), & *San Jiao Shu* (Bl 22), treat each of these with needles. (*Zhong Hua Zhen Jiu Xue [The Study of Chinese Acupuncture-moxibustion]*)

7. *Bai dai*: Commonly used points: *Dai Mai* (GB 26), *San Yin Jiao* (Sp 6), & *Qi Hai* (CV 6). Auxiliary points: *Xing Jian* (Liv 2), *Yin Ling Quan* (Sp 9), *Guan Yuan* (CV 4), & *Zu San Li* (St 36). Formula method: Use moderate stimulation. One may either not retain the needles or retain them for 15 minutes. Treat one time every other day. 10 treatments equal one course. If qi and blood are vacuous and weak, it is okay to add *Guan Yuan* and *Zu San Li*. If damp heat is pouring downward, it is okay to add *Xing Jian* and *Yin Ling Quan*. It is also alright to additionally use electroacupuncture at a moderate frequency for 5-10 minutes directed at the points on the front of the body, not the points on the extremities. (*Shang Hai Yi Xue Yuen Zhen Jiu Xue [The Shanghai College of Chinese Medicine's Study of Acupuncture-moxibustion]*)

8. *Bai dai*: First formula, use *Guan Yuan* (CV 4) & *San Yin Jiao* (Sp 6). Second formula, use *Qi Hai* (CV 6), *Gui Lai* (St 29), & *Fu Liu* (Ki 7). Third formula, use *Zi Gong* (extra point) & *Zhong Ji* (CV 3). In all three formulas use moderate stimulation. Ten days equal one course of treatment. (*Chang Yong Xin Yi Liao Fa Shou Ce [A Handbook of Commonly Used Treatments in New Medicine]*)

9. *Dai xia*: Treat by fortifying the spleen and transforming dampness or clearing heat and seeping dampness assisted by regulating and disinhibiting the *chong* and *ren*. Points to choose from: *Guan Yuan* (CV 4), *Dai Mai* (GB 26), & *San Yin Jiao* (Sp 6). If the color is white, add *Qi Hai* (CV 6) & *Yin Ling Quan* (Sp 9). If the color is yellow, add *Yin Bai* (Sp 1), *Zu San Li* (St 36) , & *Xing Jian* (Liv 2). If the color is red, add *Jian Shi* (Per 5). (*Zhen Jiu Xue Jian Bian [A Concise Study of Acupuncture-moxibustion]*)

The foregoing excerpts from premodern and contemporary Chinese texts should give English-speaking practitioners of Chinese medicine a much fuller and more complete understanding of the causes, mechanisms, diagnosis, and treatment of *dai xia*. In addition, they will also hopefully provide a better understanding of the theoretical evolution of TCM as a style of Chinese medicine.

Vaginitis
Yin Dao Yan

Vaginitis is called *yin dao yan* in the Chinese medical literature. *Yin* is the same *yin* as in *yin yang*. The vagina is one of the *er yin* or two yin in women, the other being the anus. It is sometimes also called the *qian yin* or front yin in contradistinction to the anus which is the rear yin. *Dao* is the same *dao* as in *Dao De Jing (Classic on the Way & Virtue)*, the famous Daoist classic attributed to Lao Zi. *Dao* means path. *Yan* means inflammation. In the modern TCM literature, disease names ending in *yan* translate Latinate disease categories ending in -itis. Therefore, *yin dao yan* literally means inflammation of the yin pathway or vagina. Vaginitis is not a traditional disease category appearing in premodern Chinese gynecology texts. This is because vaginal lesions were often categorized as a subdivision of *wai ke* or external medicine, whereas gynecology was classically considered a subdivision of *nei ke* or internal medicine. Because abnormal vaginal discharge (*dai xia*) typically accompanies most cases of vaginitis, most older Chinese gynecology texts discuss vaginitis under the category *dai xia*. However, under the influence of modern Western medicine, many contemporary Chinese gynecology texts now discuss vaginitis separately under the heading of *yin dao yan*.

Premodern Categories of Vaginal Disease

Before immediately presenting the modern TCM discussion of vaginitis, I would like to present a more traditional discussion of vaginal diseases found in *Yi Zong Jin Jian (The Golden Mirror of Ancestral Medicine)*, the most famous Qing dynasty compendium of Chinese medicine edited by Wu Qian and published in 1742 CE. In the section titled "Secret Tricks of the Trade of Gynecology," there is a subsection titled "Chapter on

Various Disorders of the Front Yin." Under this heading, the authors of the *Yi Zong Jin Jian* discuss nine different vaginal pathologies.

The first vaginal pathology discussed in the *Yi Zong Jin Jian* is *yin zhong* or swollen vagina. "Swelling and distention with either a dragging pain in the fetal door (another name for the vagina) or a bearing down, achy pain is called *hong xuan*." It is due to effulgent fire in the two channels of the liver and heart and damp heat flowing down into the vagina. For this condition, use *Long Dan Xie Gan Tang* (Gentiana Drain the Liver Decoction). If it is caused by habitual vacuity of the central qi, patients will feel a dragging weight in the lower abdomen. In this case, use *Bu Zhong Yi Qi Tang* (Supplement the Center & Boost the Qi Decoction). Externally, one can use *Qi Ai Fang Feng Da Ji Ao Tang* (Artemesia, Ledebouriella & Euphorbia Seu Knoxia Decoction) as a fumigant and wash. This is made by taking one handful of Folium Artemisiae Argyii (*Ai Ye*) from Qizhou in Hubei and 9 grams each of Radix Ledebouriellae Divaricatae (*Fang Feng*) and Radix Euphorbiae Seu Knoxiae (*Da Ji*) and decocting these in water. The patient then squats over the steaming decoction exposing their external genitalia directly to the steam arising from it. As the decoction cools down, the external genitalia are then also washed with this liquid. Furthermore, one can also use a powder made from equal amounts of Fructus Immaturus Citri Aurantii (*Zhi Shi*) and Pericarpium Citri Reticulatae (*Chen Pi*) which have been stir fried. This paste is applied to the affected area and the authors say that it will immediately relieve the swelling and, therefore, automatically relieve the pain.

The second vaginal pathology discussed in the *Yi Zong Jin Jian* is *yin tong* or vaginal pain. Pain inside the vagina is also called colloquially small household marriage pain. This makes me think that the pain being described is due to loss of virginity. However one Chinese doctor I queried on this said that it is simply a folk name for vaginal pain in northern China. The pain may frequently be so extreme that the patient is unable to stretch their hands and feet. This suggests someone curled up in a ball in intense pain. The cause is given as evil heat injuring the liver and spleen and damp heat pouring downward into the vagina. The authors say that *Xiao Yao San Jia Dan Pi Zhi Zi* (Rambling Powder with Moutan

& Gardenia) is appropriate to take internally. Externally, one may use the ingredients of *Si Wu Tang* (Four Materials Decoction) which are powdered and mixed with Resina Olibani (*Ru Xiang*). The resulting mass is shaped into a round, flat cake and inserted inside the vagina. This will immediately calm the pain according to Wu Qian *et al.*

Yin yang or vaginal itching is the third category of vaginal pathology discussed in the *Yi Zong Jin Jian*. Due to damp heat, *chong* or parasites arise. Typically this condition is accompanied by physical fatigue and dribbling urination. The appropriate formulas to be considered are *Xiao Yao San* (Rambling Powder) and *Long Dan Xie Gan Tang* (Gentiana Drain the Liver Decoction). Externally, one may use a combination of Semen Pruni Persicae (*Tao Ren*) ground up into a paste and mixed with powdered Realgar (*Xiong Huang*). One then takes a piece of chicken liver, slices it open, and sprinkles this paste inside the liver. Then one inserts the piece of liver into the vagina. According to the authors of the *Yi Zong Jin Jian*, the *chong* or parasites, smelling the meaty aroma of the liver, will dive into it to suck and eat it. When the liver is pulled out of the vagina, the disease is instantly cured.

The fourth vaginal pathology is *yin ting*. *Ting* means something sticking out. *Yin ting* refers to a second or third degree prolapsed uterus. According to Wu Qian *et al.*, *yin ting* is due to injury and damage to the *bao luo*, the network vessels linking the kidneys to the uterus. It may also be due to extreme efforting during childbirth, prolapse of vacuous qi, or damp heat pouring downward. In *yin ting*, a substance protrudes from within the vagina which looks like a snake, a mushroom, or a chicken's coxcomb. In ancient times, this condition was called *lai shan* or bald hernia. This name is descriptive of uterine prolapse which is more commonly called *zi gong tuo chui* (fetal palace falling downward). Modern Chinese gynecology texts, such as *Zhong Yi Fu Ke Shou Ce (A Handbook of Chinese Gynecology)* list the etiologies of uterine prolapse as damp heat pouring downward, central qi falling downward, and blood vacuity.

If the patient has swelling and pain and frequent, red urination, they belong to the heat category. For these patients, *Long Dan Xie Gan Tang* (Gentiana Drain the Liver Decoction) is appropriate. If the patient has a heavy, sagging feeling in their lower abdomen and their urine is clear and long, then they belong to the vacuity category. For these patients, *Bu Zhong Yi Qi Tang Jia Qing Pi Zhi Zi* (Supplement the Center & Boost the Qi Decoction with Green Orange Peel & Gardenia) is appropriate. For external use, use Fructus Cnidii Monnieri (*She Chuang Zi*), 15g, and Fructus Pruni Mume (*Wu Mei*), 9 pieces. Decoct these in water and use as a fumigant and wash. This same formula is given in *Zhong Yi Fu Ke Shou Ce* for the external treatment of specifically damp heat in the liver channel uterine prolapse. Following this, mix powdered Herba Chenopodii Albi (*Tu Jing Jie*) with lard and apply to the affected area. Wu Qian *et al.* say there is no one who cannot be cured by this. Chenopodium is used for skin lesions due to worms or parasites.

Yin chuang means vaginal ulcers or sores. According to the authors of the *Yi Zong Jin Jian*, these are caused by small parasites which corrode the inside of the vagina. However, the internal etiology which gives rise to the ground upon which these parasites may flourish is evil fire due to the seven passions damaging the liver and spleen, qi and blood congelation and stagnation, and damp heat pouring downward. If these conditions endure, parasites arise. The signs and symptoms of this condition are open sores which exude a watery discharge, some aching, and some itching. All of these suggest parasitic activity. In addition, the lower abdomen may be full and distended, the urination red and frequent, the appetite poor, and the body fatigued. There may also be internal heat and tidal fever, irregular menstruation, and red and white *dai xia*.

Treatment of this condition should be based on differential diagnosis. If there is swelling and pain, use *Si Wu Tang* (Four Materials Decoctiion) with Radix Bupleuri (*Chai Hu*), Fructus Gardeniae Jasminoidis (*Zhi Zi*), and Radix Gentianae Scabrae (*Long Dan Cao*). If there are festering sores with watery discharge and pain, use *Jia Wei Xiao Yao San* (Added Flavors Rambling Powder, *i.e.* Rambling Powder with Moutan & Gardenia). And if there is aching and a sagging feelings in the lower abdomen, use *Bu Zhong Yi Qi Tang* (Supplement the Center & Boost the Qi Decoction). Wu Qian *et al.* do not give any external treatments for this condition.

Yin Dao Yan/Vaginitis

The sixth category of vaginal pathologies discussed in the *Yi Zong Jin Jian* is *yin zhi* or vaginal piles. As Wu Qian *et al.* say, meat projecting out of the vagina is called vaginal piles. The common name for this condition amongst the Chinese folk is eggplant disease. This common name describes the shiny, purplish, rounded appearance of piles or hemorrhoids. If there is a yellow, watery discharge, Wu Qian *et al.* consider this condition relatively easy to treat. If instead there is a white, watery discharge, the condition is difficult to treat. Externally, use aged Radix Aconiti (*Wu Tou*) stewed in strong vinegar to fumigate the affected area. This will immediately benefit this condition. Internally, take either *Xiao Yao San* (Rambling Powder), *Bu Zhong Yi Qi Tang* (Supplement the Center & Boost the Qi Decoction), or *Gui Pi Tang* (Restore the Spleen Decoction) depending upon whether the case is one of vacuity or repletion.

The seventh category of vaginal pathology given in this Qing dynasty compendium is *yin leng*. Literally this means vaginal chill. However, this also means female frigidity or lack of sexual desire. According to Wu Qian *et al.*, most cases of *yin leng* are caused by wind cold taking advantage of vacuity and thus settling in the fetal viscus. In addition, it may also be due to enduring blood stasis and stagnant qi. Mostly it is due to a transformation of some other condition or due to enduring difficulty in pregnancy. In most cases, *Gui Fu Di Huang Wan* (Cinnamon & Aconite Rehmannia Pills, aka *Jin Gui Shen Qi Wan* or *Ba Wei Di Huang Wan*) are suitable. Externally, use equal amounts of finely powdered Radix Polygalae Tenuifoliae (*Yuan Zhi*), dry Rhizoma Zingiberis (*Gan Jiang*), Fructus Cnidii Monnieri (*She Chuang Zi*), and Fructus Evodiae Rutecarpae (*Wu Zhu Yu*). Wrap this powder in fine silk and insert into the vagina. Cure should be easy in two days.

Yin chui means vaginal flatulence.[6] Some women's vaginas habitually emit air which makes a sound. This gas comes from the grain, *i.e.*,

---

[6] Many Chinese gynecology texts, including contemporary ones, discuss this disease category. I have only seen one case in 20 years. It has been suggested to me that a predilection for a female's inverted body position (similar to the yoga posture called "The Plow") during intercourse may result in the concern over this condition.

intestinal, tract or pathway. According to the *Jin Gui Yao Lue (Essentials from the Golden Cabinet)*, grain qi repletion causes stomach qi to discharge downward. For this condition, one may use *Gao Fa Jian* (Fat Emission Decoction). *Gao Fa Jian* is first recorded in Zhang Zhong-qing's *Jin Gui Yao Lue*. Zhang likewise says this formula treats downward discharge of stomach qi which results in "breaking wind with a continuous loud sound from the vagina." This formula is made by melting a handful of woman's hair in pork fat and drinking this. According to Wu Qian *et al.*, this will conduct the disease out of the body via the urination and is an extremely effective remedy. Zhang Zhong-qing, on the other hand, says the grain qi will be conducted out through the rectum as normal flatulence. If qi and blood are greatly vacuous and the central qi has fallen downward, *Shi Quan Da Bu Tang* (Ten [Ingredients] Completely & Greatly Supplementing Decoction) with Rhizoma Cimicifugae (*Sheng Ma*) and Radix Bupleuri (*Chai Hu*) is suitable to lift what has fallen.

The last category of vaginal pathology discussed in the *Yi Zong Jin Jian* is called *jiao jie chu xue zheng*. Literally this means conjunction bleeding disorder. This means vaginal bleeding due to sexual intercourse. According to Wu Qian *et al.*, frequent vaginal bleeding with union is most often caused by damage and detriment to the heart and spleen. Therefore, *Gui Pi Tang* (Restore the Spleen Decoction) with Terra Flava Usta (*Fu Long Gan*) is suitable to take internally. According to Sun Si-miao in the *Qian Jin Yao Fang (Essential Formulas [Worth] a Thousand [Pieces of] Gold)*, one may also use Cortex Cinnamomi Cassiae (*Rou Gui*) and black soot from the bottom of cooking pots. Equal amounts of these two ingredients should be powdered and mixed with wine. One takes one spoonful of this mixture at a time and Wu Qian *et al.* considered this remedy quite effective.

Contemporary Discussion of Vaginitis

In contradistinction to the very traditional discussion of vaginal pathologies given above, Sung Jia-ling, the author of *Fu Ke Zheng Zhi (Gynecology Patterns & Treatments)*, published in Hebei in 1983, begins his discussion of vaginitis by saying that it is most often a combination of internal and external etiologies. Its internal cause is long-term pent-up liver qi transforming into heat, typically complicated by an vacuous spleen not moving fluids. When body fluids stop flowing, they gather and accumulate and transform into dampness. Liver heat and spleen dampness become mutually entangled and pour downward below, invading and soaking the vagina. With the passing of time, toxic evils are usually engendered internally. The external causes of vaginitis mostly have to do with poor vaginal hygiene and toxic evils. Evil toxins burn and damage the vagina causing inflammation.

Modern TCM gynecology texts typically divide vaginitis into three distinct patterns. These are trichomonas vaginitis, hemophilus vaginitis, and senile vaginitis. These are modern Western medical disease categories and typify the integration of modern Western and traditional Chinese diagnoses in contemporary TCM. According to *The Merck Manual*, *Trichomonas vaginalis* is a flagellated protozoan found in the genito-urinary tract of both sexes and is a common cause of vaginitis. What the Chinese refer to as hemophilus is more commonly known in the West as genital candidiasis or yeast infection.[7] Most Western clinicians are aware of the growing incidence of candida infections in the American female population due to the use of broad-spectrum antibiotics, oral contraceptives and corticosteroids, and poor dietary practices. Usually such vaginal candidiasis is due to migration of this yeast from the intestines. Senile vaginitis due to the decline of estrogen and progesterone levels in postmenopausal women is also called atrophic vaginitis. Although pathogenic microbes may be present, their presence and proliferation is a function of immune depression in turn due to humoral imbalance. In addition to these three kinds of vaginitis, modern Western medicine also

---

[7] There seems to be a problem here with the Chinese terminology. Hemophilus vaginitis and vaginal candidiasis are two different conditions. The Chinese literature all say the pattern name is hemophilus, but then they go on to discuss *Candida albicans* as the offending disease cause.

identifies vaginitis due to gardnerella, chlamydia, and herpes infection, and vaginitis due to local abscess.[8]

1) Trichomonas Vaginitis

Disease Causes: This is caused by infection by *Trichomonas vaginalis*.

Signs & Symptoms: Typically there is a yellow vaginal discharge which is spongy and frothy in consistency. It may also be similar to rice-washing water, *i.e.*, cloudy or turbid. It is accompanied by a foul smell. There is intense vaginal itching which is difficult to bear. Urination is short and reddish. Microscopic examination reveals trichomoniasis.

Therapeutic Principles: Clear heat and disinhibit dampness, kill parasites and stop vaginal discharge

Guiding Prescription: *Wu Mei Yin Chen Tang* (Mume & Capillaris Decoction)

Fructus Pruni Mume (*Wu Mei*), 30g
Fructus Zanthoxyli Bungeani (*Chuan Jiao*), 9g
Flos Lonicerae Japonicae (*Jin Yin Hua*), 12g
Herba Artemisiae Capillaris (*Yin Chen Hao*), 15g
Herba Polygoni Avicularis (*Bian Xu*), 9g
Sclerotium Poriae Cocos (*Fu Ling*), 15g
Rhizoma Atractylodis (*Cang Zhu*), 9g
Cortex Phellodendri (*Huang Bai*), 9g
Radix Gentianae Scabrae (*Long Dan Cao*), 9g

---

[8] For a discussion of the Chinese diagnosis and treatment of chlamydia vaginitis, please see the Blue Poppy Recent Research Report on this disease.

Cook the above medicinals twice in two separate batches of water. Then combine the resulting decoctions and divide into three equal portions. Take one portion three times per day. Take repeatedly for seven days.

External Wash:

Radix Sophorae Flavescentis (*Ku Shen*), 30g
Fructus Cnidii Monnieri (*She Chuang Zi*), 30g
Radix Stemonae (*Bai Bu*), 15g
Rhizoma Coptidis Chinensis (*Huang Lian*), 9g
Radix Euphorbiae Helioscopiae (*Ze Qi*), 6g

Decoct and use both as a fumigant and a wash. In other words, the patient should squat over the steaming decoction exposing their genitalia to the steam rising off it. After the liquid has cooled to be bearable to the skin, the genitalia should be washed with this decoction. This should be repeated once each morning and night for seven consecutive days.

Vaginal Suppository: *Xiong She Wan* (Realgar & Cnidium Pills)

Realgar (*Xiong Huang*), 3g
Fructus Cnidii Monnieri (*She Chaung Zi*), 9g

Finely grind the above two ingredients together and make into pills with honey each weighing three grams. Wrap each pill well in gauze and tie with a string in the middle so that a length of string one foot long hangs off. This is to enable this pill's removal. Every day, do the above fumigation and wash. Before going to sleep at night, insert one pill inside the vagina. The next morning remove. Repeat this procedure for seven days.

2) Hemophilus Vaginitis

Disease Causes: This is due to infection by *Candida albicans*. It frequently occurs in pregnant women, diabetics, those who wear the same under garments for a long time without washing, and those who habitually use antibiotics.

Signs & Symptoms: The vaginal discharge is milky white in color and lumpy in shape like tofu dregs (*i.e.*, curdy). There is itching and burning heat from the vagina to the outer genitalia, achy pain which does not diminish with pressure, and also yellowish urination. Microscopic examination reveals fungal hyphae.

Therapeutic Principles: Clear heat and resolve toxins, disinhibit dampness and stop vaginal discharge

Guiding Prescription: *Long Dan Xie Gan Tang Jia Jian* (Gentiana Drain the Liver Decoction with Additions & Subtractions)

Radix Gentianae Scabrae (*Long Dan Cao*), 9g
Radix Scutellariae Baicalensis (*Huang Qin*), 9g
Cortex Phellodendri (*Huang Bai*), 9g
Fructus Gardeniae Jasminoidis (*Zhi Zi*), 9g
Rhizoma Atractylodis (*Cang Zhu*), 12g
Fructus Kochiae Scopariae (*Di Fu Zi*), 15g
uncooked Radix Rehmanniae (*Sheng Di*), 15g
Caulis Akebiae (*Mu Tong*), 9g
Semen Plantaginis (*Che Qian Zi*), 15g

Make and take the same way as the guiding prescription given above under trichomoniasis.

External Wash:

Fructus Cnidii Monnieri (*She Chuang Zi*), 30g
Radix Sophorae Flavescentis (*Ku Shen*), 30g
Cortex Phellodendri (*Huang Bai*), 15g
Fructus Zanthoxyli Bungeani (*Chuan Jiao*), 9g
Alumen (*Ku Fan*), 9g
Cortex Radicis Dictamni Dasycarpi (*Bai Xiang Pi*), 15g

Decoct and use both as a fumigant and as a wash once per day. One course of treatment is 10 days.

Vaginal Suppository:

powdered Concha Meretricis (*Hai Ge Ke*), 30g
Borneolum (*Bing Pian*), 3g
Realgar (*Xiong Huang*), 16g

Grind the above ingredients together into a powder and mix with roasted sesame oil to form a paste. Rinse the vagina with a 4% carbonic acid sodium water solution. Then apply the above herbal paste directly to the affected area.

3) Senile Vaginitis

Disease Causes: Due to the decline in ovarian function in older women, female hormone levels drop. This results in the skin of the upper vagina becoming brittle and flimsy. Glycogen is also reduced and the acid nature of the vagina declines. This results in the immune resistance of this organ declining and becoming insufficient, thus permitting germs to breed and multiply. Menstruation, with its fluctuations in hormone levels, plays a part and, as it approaches, there appears inflammation.

Signs & Symptoms: There is a burning, scorching sensation in the vagina. There is also itching from the genitalia. Vaginal discharge is excessive. Its color is yellow and may be pussy in nature. It may also be simultaneously red and white. Gynecologic examination reveals a sticky, gluey vagina which is moist and red. There may be possible breakthrough bleeding or spotting or bleeding with intercourse. There may also be dizziness and vertigo, heart palpitations, and tinnitus. The patient's heart is easily vexed and they are easily irritable. Their tongue is red with scanty fur, and their pulse is bowstring, fine, and rapid.

Therapeutic Principles: Enrich yin and downbear fire, clear heat and disinhibit dampness

Guiding Prescription: *Zhi Bai Di Huang Wan Jia Jian* (Anemarrhena & Phellodendron Rehmannia Pills with Additions & Subtractions)

uncooked Radix Rehmanniae (*Sheng Di*), 15g
Cortex Radicis Moutan (*Dan Pi*), 9g
Fructus Corni Officinalis (*Shan Zhu Yu*), 15g
Rhizoma Alismatis (*Ze Xie*), 9g
Sclerotium Poriae Cocos (*Fu Ling*), 9g
Radix Dioscoreae Oppositae (*Shan Yao*), 15g
Rhizoma Anemarrhenae Aspheloidis (*Zhi Mu*), 9g
Cortex Phlellodendri (*Huang Bai*), 9g
Rhizoma Smilacis Glabrae (*Tu Fu Ling*), 30g
Flos Lonicerae Japonicae (*Jin Yin Hua*), 12g
Radix Rubrus Paeoniae Lactiflorae (*Chi Shao*), 9g

Make and take as above.

External Wash:

Radix Sophorae Flavescentis (*Ku Shen*), 30g
Fructus Cnidii Monnieri (*She Chuang Zi*), 30g
Herba Mercurialis Leiocarpae (*Tou Gu Cao*), 30 g
Radix Glycyrrhizae (*Gan Cao*), 12g
Herba Taraxaci Mongolici Cum Radice (*Pu Gong Ying*), 15g
Radix Rubrus Paeoniae Lactiflorae (*Chi Shao*), 9g

Decoct in water and use as a fumigant and wash once per day. Ten days equal one course of treatment.

Shi Cheng-han, author of *Zhong Yi Fu Ke (Chinese Gynecology)* published in Beijing in 1989, divides senile vaginitis into two different patterns in contradistinction to Sun Jiu-ling above. In *Zhong Yi Ku Ke*, senile vaginitis is subdivided into yang vacuity cold damp pattern and yin vacuity damp heat pattern.

A) Yang Vacuity Cold Damp Pattern

Disease Causes: The signs and symptoms of this pattern occur because of spleen- kidney yang vacuity. This decline in source warmth leads to an inability of the *ren* and *dai mai* to astringe and secure. This then results in excessive menstruation, white *dai xia*, and the accumulation of damp evils below.

Signs & Symptoms: Excessive, pale-colored menstruation, profuse, white, watery vaginal discharge, low back pain, fatigue and lack of strength, fear of cold, cold hands and feet, dizziness and vertigo, loose stools, excessive night-time urination, a pale tongue, and a soft or soggy, fine pulse

Therapeutic Principles: Warm and supplement the spleen and kidneys, warm and transform cold and dampness

Empirical Prescription:

Herba Epimedii (*Xian Ling Pi*), 9g
Rhizoma Curculiginis Orchioidis (*Xian Mao*), 9g
Radix Angelicae Sinensis (*Dang Gui*), 9g
Fructus Lycii Chinensis (*Gou Qi Zi*), 9g
Radix Dioscoreae Oppositae (*Shan Yao*), 12g
Radix Codonopsitis Pilosulae (*Dang Shen*), 12g
Sclerotium Poriae Cocos (*Fu Ling*), 12g
Fructus Rubi Chingii (*Fu Pen Zi*), 9g

2) Yin Vacuity Damp Heat Pattern

Disease Causes: Although the senile vaginitis as described in *Fu Ke Zheng Zi* above is due to yin vacuity and damp heat as evidenced by the therapeutic principles given, the author of that text does not simply state that. Whereas, the author of *Zhong Yi Fu Ke* does. According to Shi Cheng-han, the disease mechanism of this pattern is due to accumulation of damp heat in the lower burner. This consumes and damages yin fluids, and this plus the natural consumption of yin due to aging gives rise to internal flaring of vacuity heat. Therefore, the patient experiences a scorching, burning feeling in her vagina. Heat forces the urine to flow under pressure. This then causes occasional pricking pain from the outer genitalia to the vagina. Occasionally, there may also be thick, gluey bleeding with urination. Yin vacuity and internal heat are responsible for all these signs and symptoms.

Signs & Symptoms: A burning feeling in the vagina, achy pain in the lower abdomen, occasional pricking pain on urination extending from the outer genitalia into the vagina, copious *dai xia*, occasional sticky, gluey blood, a sunken, small, rapid pulse, thin, yellow tongue fur, a glossy, peeled tongue tip, and a red tongue body proper

Therapeutic Principles: Enrich the kidneys and supplement yin, clear heat and drain fire

Typical Prescription: *Zhi Bai Di Huang Wan Jia Wei* (Anemarrhena & Phellodendron Rehmannia Pills with Added Flavors)

uncooked Radix Rehmanniae (*Sheng Di*), 12g
Radix Albus Paeoniae Lactiflorae (*Bai Shao*), 9g
Radix Dioscoreae Oppositae (*Shan Yao*), 12g
Rhizoma Alismatis (*Ze Xie*), 9g
Cortex Radicis Moutan (*Dan Pi*), 9g
saltwater stir-fried Cortex Phellodendri (*Huang Bai*), 9g
saltwater stir-fried Rhizoma Anemarrhenae Aspheloidis (*Zhi Mu*), 9g
aged Fructus Corni Officinalis (*Shan Zhu Yu*), 9g
Sclerotium Poriae Cocos (*Fu Ling*), 9g
carbonized Radix Sanguisorbae (*Di Yu*), 9g
Cortex Ailanthi Altissimae (*Chun Gen Bai Pi*), 9g

Zhong Yi Fu Ke also gives a formula for use as an external wash and fumigant. It is identified only as a "simple, easy formula."

Flos Chrysanthemi Indici (*Ye Ju Hua*), 30g
Herba Violae Yedoensitis Cum Radice (*Zi Hua Di Ding*), 30g
Herba Scutellariae Barbatae (*Ban Zhi Lian*), 30g

Fructus Cnidii Monnieri (*She Chuang Zi*), 30g
Radix Sophorae Flavescentis (*Ku Shen*), 30g

Decoct the above medicinals and use as a fumigant and wash 1-2 times per day. Ten days equal one course of treatment.

Han Bai Ling on Vaginal Itching

One further discussion of the Chinese medical diagnosis and medicinal treatment of vaginitis comes from Han Bai-ling's *Bai Ling Fu Ke (Bai Ling's Gynecology)*. Old Doctor Han does not discuss *yin dao yan* as such but rather addresses *yin yang* (vaginal itching) and vaginal parasites.

Dr. Han says that, in women, either the inside or the outside of the vagina may itch and erode.[9] On the outside, itching may be accompanied by erosion and a yellow liquid exudate. While on the inside of the vagina, there may also be erosion and itching. This condition is due to arisal of *chong* or parasites within the vagina.

In terms of etiological factors, Dr. Han mentions that impetuous and excessive anger can give rise to liver channel evil heat. When this is combined with an insatiable desire to eat uncooked or chilled foods, this causes the mutual wrestling of damp heat and dampness due to spleen vacuity. If turbid dampness does not transform and yin dampness dwells for a long time in this area, damp evils will infringe upon and enter the uterus. During the menses and post partum when the *bao mai* is vacuous and empty, infection may occur due to a combination of toxic evils and pathogenic parasites.

Han Bai-ling then goes on to quote Xu Chun-fu who says:

---

[9] Western physicians believe that internal vaginal itching is a physical impossibility, since there are no itch-sensitive nerves within the vagina itself.

Women's vaginal itch is mostly due to parasitic erosion of that area. Its initial cause is unending damp heat in which terrain arises the three worms which live inside the intestines and the stomach. This parasitic erosion makes the vaginal orifice itch. As a rule, such itching and pain is ceaseless with the local area becoming sodden and extremely swollen. In virgins and widows ... this is mostly caused but unsatisfied sexual desire and the constant dwelling on wanton thoughts. This results in congelation occurring between the anus and vagina. Accumulated and pent-up damp heat which has not been dispersed for a long time gives rise to the three worms which then cause this disease. This condition may also be caused by excessive sexual intercourse resulting in heat obstruction which causes swelling, itch, and pain inside and outside and allows an opportunity for toxins. There are no other causes (of this condition) than desire, sex, damage, and depletion.

1. Damp Heat Pouring Downward

Signs & Symptoms: Itching and pain of both the outside and inside of the vagina which is difficult to bear, some yellow, watery exudate, heart vexed and not peaceful, oral thirst, dry throat, vexation and fullness within the chest, face and tongue both red, yellow tongue fur, a preference for cold drinks, hot hands, feet, and heart, dry stools, short, reddish urination, yellow *dai xia* which is smelly and purulent, and a rapid, slippery pulse

Therapeutic Principles: Clear heat, disinhibit dampness, and resolve toxins

Foundation or Guiding Formula: *Bei Xie Shen Shi Tang* (Dioscorea Hypoglauca Seep Dampness Decoction)

Rhizoma Dioscoreae Hypoglaucae (*Bei Xie*), 9g
Semen Coicis Lachryma-jobi (*Yi Yi Ren*), 9g
Cortex Phellodendri (*Huang Bai*), 6g
Sclerotium Rubrum Poriae Cocos (*Fu Ling*), 9g
Cortex Radicis Moutan (*Dan Pi*), 9g
Rhizoma Alismatis (*Ze Xie*), 6g
Caulis Akebiae (*Mu Tong*), 6g

Talcum (*Hua Shi*), 9g

In order to seep dampness, clear heat, and resolve toxins, add:

Herba Aloes (*Lu Hui*), 3g
Rhizoma Atractylodis (*Cang Zhu*), 9g
Rhizoma Anemarrhenae Aspheloidis (*Zhi Mu*), 9g
Radix Scutellariae Baicalensis (*Huang Qin*), 9g

Alternate Formula: *Long Dan Xie Gan Tang* (Gentiana Drain the Liver Decoction)

Clinical use employ: *Zhu Yuan Fang* (Control the Origin Formula) which is made with:

Fructus Carpesii Abrotanoidis (*Hei Shi*), 9g
Pasta Ulmi Macrocarpi (*Wu Yi*), 9g
Radix Sophorae Flavescentis (*Ku Shen*), 9g

This formula (presumably for external application) is in order to kill the parasites and resolve toxins. This formula may be used when there is visible damp heat of the liver channel at the vaginal orifice.

2. Toxic Evil Infection

Signs & Symptoms: Pain and itching both inside and outside the vagina which is difficult to bear, some watery, yellow exudate, possible bloody fluid exudate, heart vexed and not peaceful, oral thirst, a preference for cold drinks, possible alternating hot and cold, inhibited defecation, stools possibly gluey and sticky, urine muddy and turbid, vagina inside swollen and distended, face and tongue both red, yellow, slimy tongue fur, and a bowstring, slow or rapid pulse

Therapeutic Principles: Clear heat, resolve toxins, and disinhibit dampness

Foundation or Guiding Formula: *Qing Re Jie Du Chu Shi Tang* (Clear Heat, Resolve Toxins & Eliminate Dampness Decoction)

uncooked Radix Rehmanniae (*Sheng Di*), 9g
Radix Scutellariae Baicalensis (*Huang Qin*), 9g
Cortex Phellodendri (*Huang Bai*), 6g
Herba Artemisiae Capillaris (*Yin Chen Hao*), 9g
Flos Lonicerae Japonicae (*Jin Yin Hua*), 12g
Fructus Forsythiae Suspensae (*Lian Qiao*), 12g
Radix Sophorae Flavescentis (*Ku Shen*), 9g
Herba Lophatheri Gracilis (*Dan Zhu Ye*), 9g
Rhizoma Coptidis Chinensis (*Huang Lian*), 9g
Radix Stemonae (*Bai Bu*), 6g
Radix Glycyrrhizae (*Gan Cao*), 6g

Medicinals for External Use: Take either fresh pork, chicken, beef, or lamb liver, about 1-2 inches, and cut down the middle. Sprinkle Realgar (*Xiong Huang*) on the inside surface of the liver and insert into the vagina keeping it in place for half a day. The worms or parasites will enter the liver and will be immediately pulled out when the liver is removed. This is essentially the same external treatment which appears in the *Yi Zong Jin Jian* for vaginal itch. The fact that such a well-known contemporary Chinese gynecologist as Han Bai-ling continues to suggest this treatment up into the 1980s suggests that, although it is somewhat gross, it must work.

As in the above discussions of vaginitis from *Fu Ke Zheng Zhi*, Han Bai-ling also emphasizes the pathological role of parasites. This is important beyond vaginitis in that it establishes the etiological significance of *Candida albicans* in TCM and further categorizes such microbial infections as *chong* or parasites.

Medicinal Wine for Vaginal Itch

I would like to give two further Chinese medical protocols for the treatment of vaginitis and vaginal itch. The first is a medicinal "wine" taken internally. It appears in *Yao Jiu Yan Fang Xuan (Selected Effective Medicinal Wine Formulas)* by Sun Weng-qi and Zhu Jun-bo. Sun and Zhu state that *Ku Shen Wei Pi Jiu* (Sophora & Hedgehog Skin Wine) is indicated for the treatment of scabies, itching of the whole body, vaginal itch, and *dai xia*. It is based on the therapeutic principles of clearing heat, resolving toxins, drying dampness, and killing parasites. Its ingredients are:

Radix Sophorae Flavescentis (*Ku Shen*), 150g
Nidus Vespae (*Feng Fang*), 15g
Corium Erinacei (*Ci Wei*, 1 skin, roasted crisp

Method of Preparation: Grind the above three ingredients together into coarse powder. Using 2.5 kg of water, cook into a decoction until 1kg of liquid remains. Remove the dregs and add 150 grams of yeast, 1.5kg of millet, and mix together. Allow this to ferment similar to making other medicinal wines. While the wine is still warm, remove the distiller's grains, decant, and store for use.

Method of Administration: Take approximately one small cup, about 10ml, of this medicinal wine before each meal.

The reason I give this formula is that those practitioners who cannot afford to stock an entire Chinese medicinal pharmacy and who also do not live near such a pharmacy may make such a "wine" which will keep for at least several years. This then may be added to appropriate acupuncture therapy.

Acupuncture & Vaginal Itch

Because most Western practitioners of TCM are primarily trained and licensed as acupuncturists, most Western readers will want to know if there are any Chinese acupuncture protocols for vaginitis and vaginal itch. The following acupuncture protocol comes from Xia Zhi-ping's *Shi Yong Zhen Jiu Tui Na Zhi Liao Xue (A Study of Practical Acupuncture-moxibustion & Tuina Treatments)* published by the Shanghai College of Chinese Medicine Press in 1990. Under the heading vaginitis, two basic patters are described: 1) damp heat pouring downward, and 2) spleen-kidney vacuity detriment. The disease causes and mechanisms are the same as described above. The recommended acupuncture formula is:

Zhong Ji (CV 3)
Yin Jiao (CV 7)
San Yin Jiao (Sp 6)

These three points clear and disinhibit damp heat and stop itching. They regulate the function of the *chong* and *ren*. This formula treats vaginitis in general. For damp heat pouring downward, add *Yin Ling Quan* (Sp 9) and *Tai Chong* (Liv 3). Use draining technique. For spleen-kidney vacuity detriment, add *Shen Shu* (Bl 23) and *Zu San Li* (St 36). In that case, use even needling technique along with moxibustion. For low back aching and pain, add *Zhi Shi* (Bl 52), *Dai Mai* (GB 26), and *Ci Liao* (Bl 32). For unbearable genital itching, add *Qu Quan* (Liv 8). It is also possible to use such points as *Guan Yuan* (CV 4), *Zhi Yin* (Bl 67), *Qi Hai* (CV 6), etc. Treat once per day, retaining the needles for 30 minutes each time. Ten treatments equal one course of therapy. Between each two courses there should be a five day rest.

Dia Xia Douche

One thing that I think is evident from most of the above herbal discussions of vaginitis is that Chinese gynecology specialists have traditionally felt it necessary to treat vaginitis with both internally administered decoctions as well as with externally applied remedies. This corroborates my own experience in treating vaginitis and vaginal itching. My own external formula for damp heat, flourishing toxins vaginitis is called *Dai Xia* Douche. It is comprised of:

Fructus Cnidii Monnieri (*She Chuang Zi*), 25g
Fructus Kochiae Scopariae (*Di Fu Zi*), 25g
Alumen (*Ku Fan*), 10g
Acacia Catechu (*Er Cha*), 10g
Borax (*Peng Sha*), 10g
Resina Myrrhae (*Mo Yao*), 5g
Vinegar, 1 Tbsp.

Indications: Vaginal itch, swelling and inflammation of the external genitalia, either yellow or white *dai*, damp heat and toxins

Method of Preparation: Cook the above solid ingredients in one quart (or liter) of water. Strain the dregs and reserve the liquid. Add the vinegar. This liquid can then be used as either a douche or a wash.

Vaginal Itching
Nu Yin Sau Yang Zheng

Vaginal itching is a commonly encountered complaint in gynecological practice. As discussed in the preceding chapter on vaginitis, vaginal itching is often only discussed in the Chinese medical literature as a symptom associated with *dai xia*. However, other Chinese gynecology texts do discuss vaginal itching as its own disease category.

The following translations are from Shi Cheng-han's *Zhong Yi Fu Ke (Chinese Gynecology)* which discusses primarily the medicinal treatment of vaginal itching and Xiao Shao-qing's *Zhong Guo Zhen Jiu Chu Fang Xue (A Study of Prescription Writing in Chinese Acupuncture-moxibustion)* which discusses its acupuncture-moxibustion treatment. I have also included supplementary material from Zhang and Zhang's *Jian Ming Zhen Jiu Zhi Liao Xue (A Study of Simple, Clear Acupuncture-moxibustion Treatments)*; the Nanjing College of Chinese Medicine's *Concise Traditional Chinese Gynecology*; Xia Zhi-ping's *Shi Yong Zhen Jiu Tui Na Zhi Liao Xue (A Study of Practical Acupuncture-moxibustion & Tuina Treatments)*; Yang Jian-bao's *Xing Bing Zheng Zhi (Venereal Diseases Patterns & Treatments)*; and from Tian Cong-huo's *Zhen Jiu Yi Xue Yan Ji (A Study of Proven Acupuncture-moxibustion Theories)*. Much of this material is similar to that which appears in the previous chapter on *dai xia*. However, its inclusion and the discussion of vaginal itching as a separate disease category should prove helpful to English-speaking practitioners of TCM.

Shi Cheng-han begins by defining vaginal itching as a disease category. Shi says vaginal itching is a single category which refers to any itching of the external genitalia in females. At its tiniest or least, it may only involve the base of the vagina or it may reach the labia minora. It may also involve the entire external genitalia, even surrounding the anus. Itching is frequently worse at night than during the day. It may affect one's sleep or even one's work.

Disease Causes & Disease Mechanisms:

TCM generally divides the causes of itching of the external genitalia into vacuity and repletion types. Owing to damp heat pouring downward or infectious disease by parasites and parasitic erosion of the inside of the vagina, itching of the external genitalia may occur. This is categorized as a replete heat pattern. Owing to chronic disease or aging, the body may become vacuous and weak. The liver and kidneys become insufficient and the essence and blood vacuous and weak. Due to blood vacuity, wind is engendered and transforms into dryness. This causes roughness and itching of the vaginal area. This is categorized as a vacuity heat pattern.

When Shi Cheng-han mentions parasites, this is an allusion to the fact that TCM recognizes trichomoniasis and candidiasis as species of parasitic infections. Owing to the nature of the Chinese language, Shi is able to juxtapose, without a verb or conjunction, the TCM disease cause and disease mechanism of damp heat pouring downward with the Western medical etiology of parasitic infection, thus implying that these two are synonymous. Shi has more to say on the Western etiology of vaginal itch below.

The external genitalia are traversed by the liver channel. According to viscera and bowel pattern discrimination, the occurrence of vaginal itching is closely related to liver channel stagnant heat or harbored damp evils pouring downward.

Western medicine thinks that the cause of itching of the external genitalia is due to either hemophilus vaginitis or trichomonas vaginitis. Senile atrophic vaginitis may also cause itching of the external genitalia. It is also possible to have tinea of the external genitalia or eczema (literally, damp rash) as well as excessive white *dai*, urinary fistula, and fecal (*i.e.*, anal) fistula, in which case it is not correct or proper to irrigate the vagina with medicinal juices which may only irritate the exterior and give rise to even more itching of the external genitalia. Further, this condition may also appear in conjunction with diabetes, vitamin A, B, and C deficiencies, and other such systemic diseases. Although only a small number of patients with this condition have such systemic diseases, one should search until one finds the cause.

Main Points in Diagnosis & Treatment:

1. In the TCM treatment of vaginal itch, one must first clearly discriminate vacuity from repletion. The replete heat pattern is categorized as damp heat pouring downward. This commonly manifests as an oozing discharge of watery fluid from the vagina, copious *dai xia*, thin in consistency and yellow in color. This should be treated by clearing and disinhibiting dampness and heat while simultaneously killing parasites. There is also the category of liver channel stagnant heat. The manifestations of this are hard to bear itching of the external genitalia, a thick, fluid discharge which is not copious, and simultaneously heart vexation, easy irritability, dizziness, upper rib-side pain, and other such signs of liver channel illness. This should be treated by coursing the liver, draining heat, and disinhibiting dampness.

The main manifestations of the vacuity heat pattern are short, hot, astringent urination, burning heat of the genitalia, an itching feeling, and simultaneously low back soreness, tinnitus, a bitter taste in the mouth and dry throat, and other such symptoms of liver-kidney vacuity disease. This should be treated by enriching yin, downbearing fire, and moistening dryness.

2. Itching of the external genitalia and *dai xia* disease frequently occur in tandem or before or after each other. Therefore, TCM treats this condition and *dai xia* disease simultaneously or together as a unit.

3. In the treatment of this condition, stress is laid on therapy applied to the exterior parts. Acupuncture treatment for vaginal itching should be administered based on disease cause pattern discrimination. When these two are employed together (*i.e.*, acupuncture and external remedies), their result is good. Nevertheless, one should be aware that the external vaginal

skin is relatively fragile and delicate. Therefore, irritating, powerful stop-itching medicinals are not able to be used on the external genitalia.

Treatment Based on Pattern Discrimination:

1. Damp Heat Pouring Downward

Symptoms: Itching of the genitalia, extreme aching and pain, continuous yellow *dai*, and simultaneously dizziness, diminished sleep, chest and rib-side pain and fullness, short, frequent urination, a red tongue with slimy, yellow fur, a dry mouth with a taste bitter, and a bowstring, rapid pulse

Analysis of Pattern Symptoms: Liver channel damp heat pours downward or infectious disease by parasites with erosion of the vaginal orifice are usually accompanied by itching and extreme aching and pain. If there is damage and detriment to the two vessels of the *ren* and *dai*, there is usually continuous yellow *dai*. The liver and gallbladder have a mutual interior-exterior relationship. Gallbladder heat causes chest and rib-side pain and fullness, a dry mouth with a bitter taste, and dizziness and diminished sleep. Heat boils water fluids, thus causing pressure on the bladder. This results in short, numerous urination. The bowstring pulse indicates evils in the liver channel and its rapidity indicates heat. The red tongue with slimy, yellow fur indicates damp heat accumulating internally.

Therapeutic Principles: Clear and disinhibit dampness and heat at the same time as killing parasites

Guiding Formula: *Long Dan Xie Gan Tang* (Gentiana Drain the Liver Decoction)

Concise Traditional Chinese Gynecology gives the following unnamed formula for the treatment of this kind of damp heat vaginal itching:

Radix Gentianae Scabrae (*Long Dan Cao*), 10g

stir-fried Rhizoma Atractylodis (*Cang Zhu*), 10g
Cortex Phellodendri (*Huang Bai*), 10g
Cortex Radicis Dictamni Dasycarpi (*Bai Xian Pi*), 10g
Fructus Carpesii Abrotenoidis (*Hei Shi*), 10g
Rhizoma Alismatis (*Ze Xie*), 10g

Shi Cheng-han notes that if there is itching of the external genitalia but *dai xia* is not profuse, this is categorized as liver channel stagnant heat for which it is appropriate to use *Dan Zhi Xiao Yao San Jia Jian* (Moutan & Gardenia Rambling Powder with Additions & Subtractions).

Clinical Prescription:

Radix Bupleuri (*Chai Hu*), 4.5g
Rhizoma Atractylodis Macrocephalae (*Bai Zhu*), 9g
Radix Glycyrrhizae (*Gan Cao*), 4.5g
Sclerotium Poriae Cocos (*Fu Ling*), 9g
Radix Angelicae Sinensis (*Dang Gui*), 9g
Radix Albus Paeoniae Lactiflorae (*Bai Shao*), 9g
Fructus Gardeniae Jasminoidis (*Zhi Zi*), 9g
Cortex Radicis Moutan (*Dan Pi*), 9g
Cortex Radicis Dictamni Dasycarpi (*Bai Xian Pi*), 9g
Herba Schizonepetae Tenuifoliae (*Jing Jie*), 9g

2. Yin Vacuity Dry Heat

Symptoms: A feeling of scorching heat in the genitalia accompanied by itching, low back soreness, tinnitus, dizziness, blurred vision, a dry mouth and parched throat, a dry tongue with scanty fur, and a fine, rapid pulse

Analysis of Pattern Symptoms: Liver-kidney yin vacuity, essence and blood dual vacuity, and blood vacuity may all give rise to wind which transforms into dryness. This results in a sensation of scorching heat in the genitalia accompanied by an itching feeling. Essence-blood insufficiency and loss of ascension of essence to the clear orifices above cause the tinnitus, dizziness, and blurred vision. Yin fluid vacuity results in dry mouth and parched throat. The low back is the mansion of the kidneys.

Therefore, kidney vacuity results in low back soreness. The red tongue with scanty fur and the fine, rapid pulse are all indications of yin vacuity and internal heat.

Therapeutic Principles: Enrich yin, downbear fire, and moisten dryness

Guiding Formula: *Zhi Bai Di Huang Wan Jia Wei* (Anemarrhena & Phellodendron Rehmannia Pills with Added Flavors) from the *Yi Zong Jin Jian (Golden Mirror of Ancestral Medicine)*

Cortex Phellodendri *(Huang Bai)*, 9g
Rhizoma Anemarrhenae Aspheloidis *(Zhi Mu)*, 9g
uncooked Radix Rehmanniae *(Sheng Di)*, 12g
Fructus Corni Officinalis *(Shan Zhu Yu)*, 9g
Radix Dioscoreae Oppositae *(Shan Yao)*, 9g
Cortex Radicis Moutan *(Dan Pi)*, 9g
Rhizoma Alismatis *(Ze Xie)*, 9g
Sclerotium Poriae Cocos *(Fu Ling)*, 9g
Radix Glycyrrhizae *(Gan Cao)*, 4.5g
Tuber Ophiopogonis Japonici *(Mai Dong)*, 9g

Note: This basic pattern commonly occurs in senile, atrophic vaginitis. There may simultaneously be liver-kidney yin vacuity with fire effulgence condition. For this, use the formula *Zhi Bai Di Huang* to nourish yin and downbear fire with the addition of Licorice and Ophiopogon to engender fluids and moisten dryness. Yang Jian-bao, in *Xing Bing Zheng Zhi (Venereal Disease Patterns & Treatments)* gives a slightly different version of *Zhi Bai Di Huang Wan* for the treatment of genital candidiasis of the liver-kidney yin vacuity type. Yang adds Cortex Radicis Dictamni Dasycarpi *(Bai Xian Pi)* and Fructus Kochiae Scopariae *(Di Fu Zi)* to the basic eight ingredients of this well known formula.

Herbal Formulas for External Use:

1. *She Chuang Zi San* (Cnidium Powder)

Fructus Cnidii Monnieri (*She Chuang Zi*)
Flos Citri Erythrocarpae (*Ju Hua*)
Alumen (*Ku Fan*)
Radix Stemonae (*Bai Bu*)
Radix Sophorae Flavescentis (*Ku Shen*), 9-15g each

Decoct with water. First take advantage of the heat to fumigate with the rising steam. Then use as a sitz bath. Do one treatment per day with 10 treatments equaling one complete course of therapy.

2. Unnamed formula

powdered Conchae Meretricis (*Hai Ge Ke*), 3g
Borneolum (*Bing Pian*), 0.3g

Grind into a fine powder. Apply this medicinal powder to the external genitalia. One can also mix this powder with roasted sesame oil and apply. Use 1-2 times per day. Ten treatments (*i.e.*, 10 days) equal one complete course of therapy. This method is suitable for eczema of the external genitalia and allergic dermatitis.

3. Decoct one whole Bulbus Allii (*Da Suan*, garlic) and use as a fumigant and wash. Ten treatments equal one complete course of therapy. This formula is effective for stopping itch and killing parasites.

Concise Traditional Chinese Gynecology gives two other unnamed formulas for external treatment although that book does not clearly state that they are to be used externally.

1. Fructus Cnidii Monnieri (*She Chuang Zi*), 10g
   Cortex Phellodendri (*Huang Bai*), 10g
   Alumen (*Ku Fan*), 6g

The authors of this book say that this formula is a specific for pruritus vulvae due to trichomonas vaginitis. The authors also say that, in the treatment of trichomonas vaginitis, it is necessary to supplement acupuncture-moxibustion with direct application of external remedies.

Acupuncture alone is not, in their opinion, an adequate treatment for this type of vaginitis.

2. Cortex Radicis Pseudolaricis (*Tu Jin Pi*), 15g
   Radix Sophorae Flavescentis (*Ku Shen*), 15g
   Borneolum (*Bing Pian*), 2g

This formula is indicated specifically for pruritus vulvae due to hemophilus vaginitis.

Acupuncture

Xiao Shao-qing, acupuncture professor at the Nanjing College of Chinese Medicine gives the following formula for the treatment of vaginal itching. It is called *Qing Re Li Shi Zhi Yang Fang* (Heat-clearing, Dampness-disinhibiting, Itch-stopping Formula).

Prescription:

Ba Liao (Bl 31-34)	drain
Guan Yuan (CV 4)	"
Zhong Ji (CV 3)	"
Xue Hai (Sp 10)	"
Wei Zhong (Bl 40)	bleed
Da Dun (Liv 1)	drain
Zhi Yin (Bl 67)	"

Indications: Genital itching, very possibly accompanied by aching and pain. The limbs and body are weary and slack, and the urination is dribbling and dripping.

Additional Points Based on Presenting Symptoms:

For heart vexation and extreme itching, add *Shao Fu* (Ht 8) and *Xing Jian* (Liv 2).

Nu Yin Sau Yang Zheng/Vaginal Itch

For damp heat pouring downward, add *Yin Ling Quan* (Sp 9) and *Bai Chong Wo* (extra point one *cun* above *Xue Hai* [Sp 10]).

Formula Rationalization: This basic formula has the effects of clearing heat, disinhibiting dampness, and stopping itch. *Ba Liao* and *Zhong Ji* are able to move the qi and disinhibit dampness. *Guan Yuan* and *Xue Hai* have the ability to clear the blood and transform dampness. *Wei Zhong* and *Da Dun* both have the ability to clear heat and harmonize the liver. And *Zhi Yin* has the virtue of precipitating dampness and turbidity.

Zhang and Zhang in *Jian Ming Zhen Jiu Zhi Liao Xue (A Study of Simple, Clear Acupuncture-moxibustion Treatments)* give the same acupuncture formula. Under the heading therapeutic principles, they state that in the treatment of vaginal itch one should mainly use points on the foot *tai yang* and *ren* to clear heat and disinhibit dampness. They also specify a *shou fa* or hand technique: Puncture with fine needle using draining technique. And in their formula rationalization, they say that *Wei Zhong* clears and drains blood heat and that it is specifically *Da Dun* which harmonizes the liver.

Verification of the Functions of These Points

1. *Ba Liao*: Made up from *Shang Liao* (Bl 31), *Ci Liao* (Bl 32), *Zhong Liao* (Bl 33), and *Xia Liao* (Bl 34), left and right, altogether eight points. These transport points directed at female genital itch have a markedly good effect. The *Lei Jing Tu Yi (The Illustrated Appendix to the Systematized Classic)* says: "*Shang Liao* treats female infertility, itching and pain inside the vagina, vaginal protrusion, red and white *dai xia*." The *Jia Yi Jing* (a.k.a. the *Zhen Jiu Jia Yi Jing, [The Systematic Classic of Acupuncture-moxibustion])* says: "An unrestrained, dark green fluid below in women, a red trickle, itching and pain within the vagina...*Xia Liao* controls [this]."

2. *Zhong Ji*: The *Jia Yi Jing* says: "Itching inside the female's *yin*...*Zhong Ji* controls [this]."

3. *Xue Hai*: The *Lei Jing Tu Yi* says: "Controls kidney treasury (*i.e.*, viscus) wind, ulcers, itching, and dampness of both legs, and unbearable dampness."

4. *Wei Zhong*: The *Zhi Liao Hui Yao (The Collected Essentials of Treatment)* says: "Needling *Wei Zhong* is not only effective for *ding* ulcer but is also effective for welling abscesses and deep-rooted ulcers which are red, swollen, achy, and painful and for wind dampness of the legs and knees, also lameness due to flogging with a cane." In the light of the fact that *Wei Zhong* is also called *Xue Xi* or Blood Cleft, needling it to bleed can clear and drain the heat toxins from the blood division. For this reason, it can be used for women's vaginal itching.

5. *Da Dun*: The *Qian Jin Fang (Formulas [Worth] a Thousand [Pieces of] Gold)* says: "For the treatments of swollen, painful vagina, moxa *Da Dun* three cones." The *Bao Ming Ji (A Collection of Life Protectors)* says: "For unbearable pain inside the head of the vagina, soldier (*i.e.*, male) mounting, (and) pain inside a woman's vagina, puncture the foot *jue yin* well point, *Da Dun*."

6. *Zhi Yin*: The *Bai Zheng Fu (The Hundreds of Diseases Prose Poem)* says: "*Zhi Yin* mostly cures slight corneal opacity and itching diseases that ache."

Appendix

1. This disease is mostly caused by damp heat which generates parasites from within the intestines and stomach and by visceral vacuity. When the viscera are vacuous, parasites stir and invade the yin gate or vagina. Modern medical theory believes that mostly this disease is caused by hemophilus and trichomonas infections.

2. Basic (acupuncture) treatment method for this disease: Choose *ren mai*, foot *tai yang*, and foot three yin channel points as the main or ruling points. Puncture using draining technique. Retain the needles for 20 minutes. Treat one time per day. Ten treatments equal one course of therapy.

The authors of *Concise Traditional Chinese Gynecology* give two different acupuncture prescriptions based on the TCM discrimination of repletion and vacuity patterns of vaginal itching. For damp heat in the liver channel, the formula is:

Zhong Ji (CV 3)	drain
Qu Gu (CV 2)	"
Li Gou (Liv 5)	"
Tai Chong (Liv 3)	"

If there is profuse vaginal discharge, add and also drain *Gui Lai* (St 29) and *Yin Ling Quan* (Sp 9).

For yin vacuity vaginal itching, the formula given is:

Da He (Ki 12)	supplement
Qu Gu (CV 2)	drain
Li Gou (Liv 5)	"
Fu Liu (Ki 7)	supplement
San Yin Jiao (Sp 6)	"

Xia Zhi-ping in *Shi Yong Zhen Jiu Tui Na Zhi Liao Fa (A Study of Practical Acupuncture-moxibustion & Tuina Treatments)* gives yet another couple of acupuncture prescriptions for itching of the external genitalia. Xia's acupuncture formula consists of:

Zhong Ji (CV 3)
Yin Lian (Liv 11)
Xue Hai (Sp 10)
Yin Ling Quan (Sp 9)
Li Gou (Liv 5)

According to Xia, these points clear heat and disinhibit dampness but also quicken the blood division. Based on the saying,

Zhi feng qian zhi zue
Xue xing feng si mie

> To treat wind, first treat the blood;
> When the blood moves, wind will be spontaneously extinguished,

This treatment stops itching. For acute cases, treatment should be given 1-2 times per day. Puncture with fine needles using draining technique. For chronic cases, treat once every other day using even needling technique. One can also treat this disease by using such points as *Qu Quan* (Liv 8), *San Yin Jiao* (Sp 6), *Zhi Yin* (Bl 67), etc.

Ear Acupuncture: Select from points such as ear *Shen Men*, Reproductive Organs, Lungs, Liver, Kidneys, etc. Puncture and retain the needles for 30 minutes. Treat one time per day with 5-10 treatments equaling one course of therapy. One can also use press needles in the ear points.

Tian Cong-huo, author of *Zhen Jiu Yi Xue Yan Ji (A Collection of Tested Acupuncture Medical Theories)*, also offers two treatments for vaginal itching. The first of these is a fine needle treatment:

Points Used:

Main Points: *Hui Yin* (CV 1), *Yin Lian* (Liv 11), and *Qu Gu* (CV 2)

Auxiliary Points: *Yin Ling Quan* (Sp 9) and *San Yin Jiao* (Sp 6)

Formula Needling Method:

Needle using even supplementing/even draining or other such moderately stimulating hand techniques. Retain the needles 5-15 minutes. Treat daily or once every other day, six treatments equaling one course of therapy.

Empirical Verification

Six cases of vaginal pruritus were treated with the above acupuncture treatment. The patients ranged in age from 45-55 years old. The disease course had lasted from 1/2-1 year in each case. After receiving the above method of treatment, all obtained obvious marked effect. In general, this treatment protocol achieves acceptable therapeutic results.

Tian's second "acupuncture" treatment is point injection therapy.

Points Used:

Chang Jiang (GV 1), *Qu Gu* (CV 2), *Huan Tiao* (GB 30), *Zu San Li* (St 36), and *San Yin Jiao* (Sp 6)

Formula Injection Method:

Inject 5ml of a solution made by adding 200 micrograms of vitamin B_{12} to 1% hydrochloric procaine. For itching of the front *yin* (*i.e.* the vagina), use *Qu Gu*. For itching of the rear *yin* (*i.e.*, the anus), use *Chang Jiang*. Treat once per day, 10 treatments equaling one course of therapy. After injecting points adjacent to the affected area 2-3 times, alternate by injecting once bilaterally *Zu San Li* or *San Yin Jiao*.

Tian Cong-huo also gives another point injection method using 1ml of vitamin B_1 combined with 0.2 milliliters of 2.5% procaine in which case *Chang Jiang* is injected once every three days, with 10 treatments equaling one course.

Empirical Verification:

Twenty-six cases were treated with injection therapy using a vitamin B_{12} solution. Twelve cases had itching inside the vagina. Six had itching of the external vagina, and eight had anal itching. The disease course had ranged from two months to as long as eight years. The number of treatments ranged from 8-30. Of these, eight cases were cured, six were markedly improved, another eight were somewhat improved, and four received no result.

Twenty-two cases received injection therapy with procaine at *Chang Jiang*. (Some of the patients had eczema of the vaginal meatus, itching of the vaginal meatus, anal itch, itching of the external genitalia, and eczema of the external genitalia.) After receiving treatment, eight were cured, 10 were markedly improved, three were somewhat improved, and only one showed no effect. This treatment often stops itching after a single treatment. Generally it is able to stop itching in 2-4 days.

Shi Cheng-han also gives an acupuncture treatment for vaginal itching. This is a water needle treatment similar to the point injection methods discussed above. Water needle (*shui zhen*) means the injection of various medicinal liquids into acupuncture points. Shi says to inject 0.5ml of a 1% procaine solution into *San Yin Jiao* (Sp 6) bilaterally and *Guan Yuan* (CV 4). Treat one time per day, with seven treatments equaling one complete course of therapy.

Inflammatory Conditions of the External Genitalia
Wai Yin Bu Yan Zheng

Bartholinitis & Vulvar Ulcers

Guo Yuan, author of *Shi Yong Zhong Xi Yi Jie He Fu Chan Ke Zheng Zhi (Practical Integrated Chinese-Western Medicine Patterns & Treatments)* published in Shanxi in 1984, includes the subcategory of inflammatory conditions of the external genitalia under the broader chapter heading of inflammatory conditions of the female reproductive tract (*nu xing sheng zhi qi yan zheng*). Under this category, Guo Yuan then further distinguishes the categories of bartholinitis (*qian ting da xian yan*) and vulvar ulcers (*wai yin kui yang*).

Bartholinitis

The greater vestibular gland is located posterior to the labia majora. It has an opening at the back of the vaginal vestibule in between the labia minora and the hymen. If there is any infection, this gland's duct may become swollen which, in turn, may result in adhesion and occlusion of this duct. In many cases, this leads to infection of the greater vestibular gland itself or to the formation of a cyst within the greater vestibular gland. When infection is present, the labia minora and majora may appear red and swollen making the orifice of the vagina look like a silkworm cocoon. This condition can cause extreme pain. If this condition is suppurant, the patient may experience a rippling sensation locally. In most cases, the abscess will rupture in 3-4 days. Once the purulent fluid is evacuated, the symptoms of this condition typically abate spontaneously.

If complete drainage after eruption occurs or there is prompt incision treatment (to lance and drain the abscess), this condition can be cured. However, if there is incomplete drainage, this may lead to chronic bartholinitis in which case there may be recurrent self-generating infection and only temporary recovery. It may also cause, frequent, acute recurrence as well. In addition, even without infection of the gland, adhesion and occlusion of this gland's duct can give rise to retention cyst of the greater vestibular gland.

Treatment

During the acute stage, the patient should be confined to bed. Hot compresses may be applied locally. Antibiotics are also recommended. If there is abscess, incision and drainage should be performed and antibiotics or herbal medicines should be given. Chinese medicinals should be used which clear heat and resolve toxins supplemented by medicinals which quicken the blood.

Flos Lonicerae Japonicae (*Jin Yin Hua*), 15g
Herba Taraxaci Mongolici Cum Radice (*Pu Gong Ying*), 15g
Rhizoma Smilacis Glabrae (*Tu Fu Ling*), 15g
Cortex Radicis Moutan (*Dan Pi*), 15g
Radix Rubrus Paeoniae Lactiflorae (*Chi Shao*), 15g
Rhizoma Corydalis Yanhusuo (*Yan Hu Suo*), 9g
Radix Bupleuri (*Chai Hu*), 1.5g

Decoct in water and administer internally.

In this formula, Lonicera, Dandelion, and Smilax clear heat and resolve toxins. Moutan and Red Peony quicken the blood. Corydalis stops pain. And Bupleurum is used as a guiding medicinal to lead the other medicinals to the liver channel which traverses the external genitalia.

In case of chronic bartholinitis, treatment should consist of either surgical excision of the gland or Chinese medicinals to quicken the blood and transform stasis.

Radix Angelicae Sinensis (*Dang Gui*), 15g
Radix Salviae Miltiorrhizae (*Dan Shen*), 15g
Radix Rubrus Paeoniae Lactiflorae (*Chi Shao*), 15g
Squama Manitis Pentadactylis (*Chuan Shan Jia*), 15g
Rhizoma Sparganii (*San Leng*), 6g
Rhizoma Curcumae Zedoariae (*E Zhu*), 6g
Radix Bupleuri (*Chai Hu*), 3g

Decoct in water and administer internally.

This formula is for quickening the blood, transforming stasis, and dispersing conglomerations and lumps.

In case of cyst of the greater vestibular gland, Guo Yuan says this should be treated surgically.

The authors of *Concise Traditional Chinese Gynecology* describe this same condition, *i.e.*, bartholinitis and cysts of the greater vestibular gland, under the heading boils of the vulva. Because this book was translated and published in China, it is impossible to know exactly what the Chinese heading was. Presumably it was *yin chuang*. The authors say this disease category corresponds to purulent vulvitis and cysts of the greater vestibular gland. According to them, the disease causes and mechanisms of this condition are liver channel damp heat and accumulation of toxins, qi stagnation and blood stasis due to external invasion of cold evils, and constitutional yang vacuity or vacuity cold. Due to these causes, static blood and phlegm dampness combine to form masses and lumps.

Differentiation:

Boils (read abscesses, ulcers, and cysts) of abrupt onset with local redness, swelling, and burning pain with possible oozing of purulent discharge accompanied by fever indicate replete heat. Persistent hard masses which are neither painful not itchy and are accompanied by emaciation suggest vacuity cold. And persistent purulent boils accompanied by offensively smelly, oozing pus imply accumulation of toxic heat and qi and blood vacuity detriment. This is a critical condition (possibly corresponding to cancer of the vulva).

1. Toxic Heat

In this condition, swelling and pain may suddenly occur on one or both sides of the vulva. This often causes difficulty walking at the onset of this disease. The swollen area may be crescent-shaped like a cocoon and typically festers within 3-5 days. This cocoon then usually bursts towards the membrane on the inner side of the labia majora, discharging thick, fetid pus. The wound generally heals in 5-7 days. However, pus may still flow periodically and this may result in the formation of a fistula. Along with the development of local signs and symptoms, typically there are fear of cold, fever, thirst, poor appetite, constipation, hesitant urination, yellow, slimy tongue fur, and a deep, rapid pulse.

2. Retention of Cold

In this case, there will be persistent, hard masses with only minimal swelling and pain and no discoloration of the surrounding skin. Prolonged boils (cysts or abscesses) may fester and bleed after scratching. The wound may remain a long time, frequently oozing pus. Systemic signs and symptoms include lassitude of the spirit, fatigue, poor appetite, heart palpitations, restlessness, a pale tongue with slightly yellow, slimy fur, and a fine, soft, weak pulse.

Treatment:

1. Toxic Heat

Therapeutic Principles: Clear heat and resolve toxins, quicken the blood and dispel stasis

Formula:
Flos Lonicerae Japonicae (*Jin Yin Hua*), 15g
Herba Taraxaci Mongolici Cum Radice (*Pu Gong Ying*), 10g
Caulis Sargentodoxae (*Hong Teng*), 15g

Squama Manitis Pentadactylis (*Chuan Shan Jia*), 10g
Resina Olibani (*Ru Xiang*), 5g
Resina Myrrhae (*Mo Yao*), 5g

2. Retention of Cold

A. Persistent Masses

Therapeutic Principles: Warm the channels and scatter cold, transform phlegm and nourish the blood

Formula:
Herba Ephedrae (*Ma Huang*), 3g
Semen Sinapis Albae (*Bai Jie Zi*), 9g
Cortex Cinnamomi Cassiae (*Rou Gui*), 3g
Gelatinum Cornu Cervi (*Lu Jiao Jiao*), 10g
Radix Glycyrrhizae (*Gan Cao*), 6g

B. Prolonged Festering Boils

Therapeutic Principles: Supplement the qi, nourish the blood, and resolve toxins

Formula:
Radix Panacis Ginseng (*Ren Shen*), 10g
Radix Astragali Membranacei (*Huang Qi*), 10g
Radix Angelicae Sinensis (*Dang Gui*), 10g
Radix Ligustici Wallichii (*Chuan Xiong*), 3g
Radix Platycodi Grandiflori (*Jie Geng*), 5g

I include this discussion from *Concise Traditional Chinese Gynecology* because it introduces the fact that phlegm nodulation may also play a part in the formation of cysts and neoplasms of the bartholin gland and that these are not solely an accumulation of static blood. This is especially the case in cysts and tumors of the bartholin gland which, other than their being palpable masses, are not accompanied by other obvious symptomology.

Vulvar Ulcers

Guo Yuan begins this discussion by saying that the cause of ulceration of the vulva is not entirely clear (at least to Western medicine).

1. Classification, Cause, & Clinical Manifestations

A. Simple vulvar ulcer: The vulva is red and swollen. The size of the ulcer may vary but is usually covered by a layer of purulent excreta. There is incessant, localized burning and itching.

According to TCM, the causative factors of this condition are basically agreed upon. Mostly it is due to damp heat pouring downward. The *Jin Gui* (a.k.a. *Jin Gui Yao Lue [Essentials from the Golden Cabinet]*) says:

> (If the) *shao yin* pulse is slippery and rapid,
> Ulcers have arisen within the vagina.
> (If the) ulcer within the vagina has ripened,
> Choose *Lang Ya Tang* to wash it with.

The *Fu Ren Liang Fang (Fine Formulas for Women)* says:

> If the *shao yin* pulse in women is slippery and rapid, there must be ulcers within the vagina. This is also called *shi*. There is pain and itching like worms crawling around. There is a watery discharge and erosion of the vagina can recur easily. This is due to vexation and depression of the heart and spleen, vacuity and weakness of the spleen and stomach, and stagnation and stasis of the qi and blood.

Xue Li-zhai, in *Jiao Zhu Fu Ren Liang Fang (Annotated Fine Formulas for Women)*, says: "Arisal of ulcers inside the female vagina, therefore [there is] seven passions depressive fire, damage and detriment of the liver and spleen, and damp heat pouring downward." This means that due to depressive heat from excesses of the seven emotions, the liver and spleen are damaged causing downward pouring of damp heat. It is this damp heat which results in the vaginal ulcers.

Essentially, all the above schools of thought hold an identical point of view, since a rapid pulse indicates heat and a slippery pulse indicates dampness. Heat is engendered because of depression and vexation of the heart and spleen. Dampness accumulates because of vacuity and weakness of the spleen and stomach. Dampness and heat mutually bind and pour downward to the genitalia. In the genitalia, they give rise to ulcers locally.

B. Syndrome of eyes, genitals, and juncture of the skin and (mucous) membranes: This condition, also called Behçet's syndrome, tends to occur in the spring. The area of the genitals feels itchy, irritated, and is ulcerous. Typically, at the same time, there is erythema nodosa of the lower limbs. In a few people, there may be iridocyclitis, and oral and/or pharyngeal ulcers may also be seen. The cause of this condition is not entirely clear as yet (in Western medicine). What is called the *hu huo* or "fox misled condition" in the *Jin Gui (Golden Cabinet)* and this are very similar to each other. The *Jin Gui* says:

> *Hu huo* resembles damage (due to) cold disease in that one feels taciturn and dull like being on the verge of sleep. (However,) the eyes are difficult to close, and one feels irritable no matter whether one lies down or sits up. When it erodes the throat, it is called *huo*. When it erodes the genitalia, it is called *hu*. One may lose their appetite completely and may even find the fragrance of food offensive. The face is changeable from time to time, (going from) red to black to white. If the erosion happens on the upper part of the body, the voice will be hoarse...If the erosion happens on the lower part of the body, the throat will feel dry...There may also be erosion of the anus...This condition's pulse is fast. There is no heat, but there is often vexation. One may remain quiet with a tendency to lie down with sweating. For the first 3-4 days, the eyes are red and bloodshot. By the seventh to eighth days, the four corners of the eyes are black.

The fact that the *Jin Gui* says to use the formulas *Gan Cao Xie Xin Tang* (Licorice Drain the Heart Decoction), *Chi Xiao Dou Dang Gui San* (Aduki Bean & Dang Gui Powder), and *Ku Shen Xi Fang* (Sophora Washing Formula) clearly indicates that this condition is categorized as dampness and heat.

2. Treatment

A. Simple vulvar ulcer: The *Jin Gui* says:

> If the *shao yin* pulse is slippery and rapid, this indicates the development of ulcer within the genitals. If the ulcer has ripened, use *Lang Ya Tang* to wash with. Take 3 *liang* of Radix Potentillae Cryptotaeniae (*Lang Ya*) and 4 *sheng* of water and cook till reduced to half a *sheng*. Use a piece of chopstick one end of which is wrapped in cotton. Dip this end into the decoction and insert the wrapped end of the chopstick into the vagina to moisten it. Do this four times per day.

The *Fu Ren Liang Fang (Fine Formulas for Women)* says:

> Ulcers arise in the vagina due to vexation and depression of the heart and spleen and vacuity and weakness of the spleen and stomach. This causes stagnation and stasis of the qi and blood. Treatment should proceed by supplementing the heart and boosting the stomach. Externally, one can use medicinal treatments for fumigating, washing, and sitz-bathing.

Bu Xin Tang (Supplementing the Heart Decoction)

Radix Panacis Ginseng (*Ren Shen*)
Sclerotium Poriae Cocos (*Fu Ling*)
Radix Peucedani (*Qian Hu*)
Rhizoma Pinelliae Ternatae (*Ban Xia*)
Radix Ligustici Wallichii (*Chuan Xiong*), 22.5g each
Pericarpium Citri Reticulatae (*Chen Pi*)
Fructus Citri Aurantii (*Zhi Ke*)
Folium Perillae Frutescentis (*Zi Su Ye*)
Radix Platycodi Grandiflori (*Jie Geng*)
dry Rhizoma Zingiberis (*Gan Jiang*)
Radix Glycyrrhizae (*Gan Cao*), 15g each
Radix Angelicae Sinensis (*Dang Gui*)
Radix Albus Paeoniae Lactiflorae (*Bai Shao*), 30g each
cooked Radix Rehmanniae (*Shu Di*), 45g

Add black Fructus Zizyphi Jujubae (*Hei Zao*), decoct, and administer internally.

Ma Huang Tang (Ephedra Decoction) Washing Formula:

Herba Ephedrae (*Ma Huang*)
Rhizoma Coptidis Chinensis (*Huang Lian*)
Fructus Cnidii Monnieri (*She Chuang Zi*), 30g each
Folium Artemisiae Argyii (*Ai Ye*), 45g
Fructus Pruni Mume (*Wu Mei*), 10 pcs

Crush the ingredients before decocting in water, remove the dregs, and wash with the resulting liquid while hot. Avoid wind chill.

TCM posits that simple vulvar ulcers are due to liver channel damp heat pouring downward. The onset of this problem can be so sudden that the time between the onset of itching to the development of the ulcer can be as short as from a few hours to 1-2 days. There is local redness and swelling with multiple ulcerations. The surface of the ulcer may be covered with a purulent coating. The local area feels so itchy it is hardly bearable. Also, the purulent exudate dribbles constantly. In this case, there is not only damp heat pouring downward, but there is also superficial wind heat stagnating the qi and blood in the epithelium. The onset of this condition is always characterized by itchiness first, followed by redness. This is categorized as a wind heat pattern. This should be treated by dispelling wind, clearing heat, and disinhibiting dampness.

Periostracum Cicadae (*Chan Tui*), 12g
Fructus Kochiae Scopariae (*Di Fu Zi*), 15g
Herba Ephedrae (*Ma Huang*), 6g
Radix Gentianae Scabrae (*Long Dan Cao*), 9g
Radix Scutellariae Baicalensis (*Huang Qin*), 9g
Flos Lonicerae Japonicae (*Jin Yin Hua*), 15g
Fructus Forsythiae Suspensae (*Lian Qiao*), 15g
Radix Et Rhizoma Rhei (*Da Huang*), 9g
Radix Glycyrrhizae (*Gan Cao*), 3g

Decoct in water and administer internally.

This formula is very effective for the early stage of simple vulvar ulcer. After administering four doses, Rhubarb can usually be omitted and Sclerotium Poriae Cocos (*Fu Ling*) and other such dampness-seeping medicinals and Radix Rubrus Paeoniae Lactiflorae (*Chi Shao*) and Radix Angelicae Sinensis (*Dang Gui*) for quickening the blood can be added. Approximately 10 doses (*i.e.*, 10 days of treatment) can cure this condition. This condition tends to occur around the spring festival. Therefore, three doses of the above formula can be taken around that time for prevention.

B. Syndrome of the eyes, genitals, and juncture of the skin and (mucous) membranes: Treatment of this condition is relatively difficult. In the gynecology department, one sees patients whose clinical manifestations include uncured ulcers of the external genitalia which have persisted over many years with irregular outbreaks. When there is an attack, extensive ulceration may appear with irregular borders. The ulcers are usually covered with a filthy, dark yellowish coating. At the base of the ulcers, raw flesh can be seen. The genital region feels burning hot, achy, and painful. This is commonly followed by erythema nodosa of the lower limbs. In a few cases, the oral membranes may also be ulcerated. As a rule, this condition does not cause fever. The body of the tongue is mostly purplish and dark. The cause of this disease is probably a combination of the three qi of wind, cold, and dampness which stagnate and obstruct the channels and network vessels and cause the blood vessels to be not free-flowing. Thus the qi and blood become stagnant and static and this causes the ulceration and festering in the area of the genitalia. However, at the initial stage or at the beginning of a recurrence, heat is typically found. In treatment, this should be dealt with separately.

Wind Damp Heat Pattern: Ulceration of the external genitalia, scorching heat, redness, and swelling, incessant dribbling of a watery discharge, itching and pain which are hard to bear. Treatment should dispel wind, clear heat, and disinhibit dampness.

Periostracum Cicadae (*Chan Tui*), 12g

Herba Ephedrae (*Ma Huang*), 6g
Fructus Kochiae Scopariae (*Di Fu Zi*), 15g
Radix Scutellariae Baicalensis (*Huang Qin*), 12g
Fructus Gardeniae Jasminoidis (*Zhi Zi*), 6g
Rhizoma Atractylodis (*Cang Zhu*), 9g
Sclerotium Poriae Cocos (*Fu Ling*), 15g
Radix Et Rhizoma Rhei (*Da Huang*), 9g
Flos Lonicerae Japonicae (*Jin Yin Hua*), 15g
Fructus Forsythiae Suspensae (*Lian Qiao*), 15g
Radix Glycyrrhizae (*Gan Cao*), 9g

Decoct in water and take. After taking four doses delete the Rhubarb (if the stools are now freely flowing).

Wind Cold Damp Pattern: Stubborn ulceration of the genitalia with frequent recurrence. The ulcerated area of the genitalia is extensive with a rough border which is dark purplish in color. Sometimes raw flesh can be seen on the surface covered by a scant, purulent coating. This is due to invasion of the genital region by the three qi of wind, cold, and dampness which cause obstruction of the channels, network vessels, and blood vessels. Due to enduring localized blood stasis, this condition is difficult to cure. Treatment should warm the channels and scatter cold, free the flow of the channels and quicken the network vessels, quicken the blood and drive away stagnation.

Ramulus Cinnamomi Cassiae (*Gui Zhi*), 9g
Radix Ledebouriellae Divaricatae (*Fang Feng*), 9g
Folium Perillae Frutescentis (*Zi Su Ye*), 9g
Cortex Cinnamomi Cassiae (*Rou Gui*), 6g
Fructus Foeniculi Vulgaris (*Xiao Hui Xiang*), 6g
Radix Angelicae Sinensis (*Dang Gui*), 15g
Radix Salviae Miltiorrhizae (*Dan Shen*), 15g
Caulis Milletiae Seu Spatholobi (*Ji Xue Teng*), 15 g
Radix Rubrus Paeoniae Lactiflorae (*Chi Shao*), 15g
Semen Pruni Persicae (*Tao Ren*), 9g
Flos Carthami Tinctorii (*Hong Hua*), 9g

Decoct in water and administer internally, one *ji* per day. This formula will not bring about instantaneous effect, but effectiveness is assured if it is taken for a long time. The emphasis of this formula is on quickening of the blood and driving away stagnation, thus) promoting the free flow of the qi and blood. Once that goal is achieved, the ulcers will be cured. If hard swelling of the local area is particularly severe, Rhizoma Sparganii (*Sang Leng*), Rhizoma Curcumae Zedoariae (*E Zhu*), Squama Manitis Pentadactylis (*Chuan Shan Jia*), etc. should be added.

Herpes Genitalia
Sheng Qi Zhi Pao Zhen

Yang Jian-bao, in *Xing Bing Zheng Zhi (Venereal Disease Patterns & Treatments)* published in Beijing in 1989, includes a discussion of *sheng qi zhi pao zhen*. *Sheng qi zhi* means reproductive organs. *Pao* means blister when it appears by itself and *zhen* means rash. However, when these two words are used together in modern Chinese medical literature, they refer to herpes. Therefore, *sheng qi zhi pao zhen* specifically refers to herpes genitalia. This sexually transmitted disease is widely disseminated amongst young and middle-aged Western adults and Western practitioners of TCM are frequently called upon to treat it.

Yang says that according to TCM, this condition is traditionally categorized under *yin chuang* (vaginal sores) and *re chuang* (hot sores).

1. Disease Causes & Disease Mechanisms

The etiology of herpes genitalia is solely the herpes virus type II (HSV II). Sexual intercourse is its main route of infectious transmission. Oral sex and anal intercourse cause herpes to occur at the corresponding body parts.

Internally there is damp heat and simultaneous affliction by toxins. Heat and toxins become bound up together and pour downward to the two yin and there erupt as genital herpes.

2. Distinguishing Characteristics of this Condition

A. Latency period: 2-24 days

B. Affected Areas: In men, herpes may easily erupt on the prepuce or foreskin or on the glans penis. It may also be situated in the groove below the crown. In females, herpes may easily erupt on the labia majora or minora, the mons veneris, the clitoris, or affect the uterine cervix. It may also erupt in the areas of the eyes, around the mouth, the throat and larynx, the breasts, and around the anus.

C. Clinical Manifestations: At the beginning, herpes erupts as a small rash. It very rapidly transforms into a small, watery ulcer. There is erythema around its base. It may change into a cluster or gathering of sores and, at first, there is only a little bit of pain. The periphery of these watery sores may turn into pussy ulcers and their shape may commonly become eroded. They may ooze liquid if the shallow lesions break open. At this point, there is typically intense aching and pain. After 15-20 days, a scab ripens and the lesion heals. Ordinarily, there will not be any scar.

D. Generalized Symptoms: Fever, headache, distention and pain. In women, this condition may be relatively light with few or no generalized symptoms.

E. Accompanying Conditions: Urinary tract inflammation, cystitis, non-bacterial encephalitis, pelvic inflammatory disease, lymphadenitis, vaginal yeast infection, etc.

F. Repeat Eruptions: Recurrent eruptions ordinarily repeat 4-8 months later.

3. Treatment Based on Pattern Discrimination

A. Wind Heat Type

Main Symptoms: At the beginning there is fever. There is tiny but fierce wind cold combined with external defensive not being secure. Herpes lesions may erupt around the two yin, the mouth, and nose. There is slight pain or an itching feeling. Simultaneously, there may be oral thirst and pain in the throat. The tongue is red and its fur is slimy and white or slimy and yellow. The pulse is floating and rapid.

Analysis of Symptoms: Wind heat begins the attack. Evil and righteous qi struggle together. This causes fever. Tiny but fierce wind cold and lack of fitness or wellness of the body periphery causes blockage of the body's skin by disease evils which erupts as herpes. Wind heat above obstructs the throat and larynx and causes the mouth to be thirsty and the throat painful.

Therapeutic Principles: Course and dispel wind and heat, clear heat and resolve toxins

Guiding Formula: *Yin Qiao San* (Lonicera & Forsythia Powder)

[Formula from Bensky & Barolet's *Chinese Herba Medicine: Formulas & Strategies*:

Flos Lonicerae Japonicae (*Jin Yin Hua*), 30g
Fructus Forsythiae Suspensae (*Lian Qiao*), 30g
Radix Platycodi Grandiflori (*Jie Geng*), 18g
Fructus Arctii Lappae (*Niu Bang Zi*), 18g
Herba Menthae Haplocalycis (*Bo He*), 18g
Semen Praeparatus Sojae (*Dan Dou Chi*), 15g
Herba Schizonepetae Tenuifoliae (*Jing Jie*), 12g
Herba Lophatheri Gracilis (*Dan Zhu Ye*), 12g
Rhizoma Phragmitis Communis (*Lu Gen*), 15-30g
Radix Glycyrrhizae (*Gan Cao*), 15g]

Formula Analysis: Lonicera and Forsythia clear heat and resolve toxins. Schizonepeta, Mentha, and Prepared Soybeans out-thrust evils and discharge them externally. Arctium, Platycodon, and Licorice resolve toxins and disinhibit the throat. Lophatherum and Phragmites clear heat and engender fluids in order to stop thirst.

B. Damp Heat Type

Main Symptoms: Herpes erupts in the area of the reproductive organs. There is burning heat and piercing pain. One feels their mouth bitter and throat dry. There is also thirst, vexation, dryness, and easy anger. Urination is repeated, frequent, short, and red. The tongue is red with slimy, yellow or thick, yellow fur. The pulse is slippery, fine, and rapid.

Analysis of Symptoms: Externally, there is invasion of toxins. Internally, there is liver-gallbladder damp heat. Heat and toxins bind together and pour downward to the two yin, causing herpes lesions. Liver-gallbladder fire flaring upward causes a bitter taste in the mouth and dry throat, vexation, dryness, and easy anger. The liver vessel connects with the genitalia. When liver channel dampness and heat pour downward, this results in the urination being frequent, repeated, short, and red.

Therapeutic Principles: Clear and disinhibit liver-gallbladder dampness and heat

Guiding Formula: *Long Dan Xie Gan Tang* (Gentiana Drain the Liver Decoction)

[Formula from Bensky & Barolet's *Chinese Herbal Medicine: Formulas & Strategies*:

Radix Gentianae Scabrae (*Long Dan Cao*), 3-9g
Radix Scutellariae Baicalensis (*Huang Qin*), 6-12g
Fructus Gardeniae Jasminoidis (*Zhi Zi*), 6-12g
Caulis Akebiae (*Mu Tong*), 3-6g
Semen Plantaginis (*Che Qian Zi*), 9-15g
Rhizoma Alismatis (*Ze Xie*), 6-12g
Radix Bupleuri (*Chai Hu*), 3-9g
uncooked Radix Rehmanniae (*Sheng Di*), 9-15g
Extremitas Radicis Angelicae Sinensis (*Dang Gui*), 6-12g
Radix Glycyrrhizae (*Gan Cao*), 3-6g]

Analysis of Formula: Gentiana drains replete fire from the liver-gallbladder and eliminates damp heat from the lower burner. Scutellaria and Gardenia are bitter and cold and drain fire. Alisma, Akebia, and Plantago assist Gentiana in clearing and disinhibiting damp heat and abducting fire through urination. Dang Gui Tails quicken the blood. Uncooked Rehmannia cools and quickens the blood and enriches yin. Bupleurum courses and soothes the liver-gallbladder, and Licorice regulates the middle and harmonizes the other medicinals.

C. External Medicinal Treatments:

Apply a 2% solution of gentian violet externally. If there are water blisters, one can use *Qing Dai Gao* (Indigo Ointment), *Si Huang Gao* (Four Yellows Ointment), etc. after these have broken open.

Qing Dai Gao (Indigo Ointment)

Pulvis Indigonis (*Qing Dai*)
powdered Cortex Phellodendri (*Huang Bai*), 20g each
Gypsum Fibrosum (*Shi Gao*)
Talcum (*Hua Shi*), 40g each

Take 25 grams of the resulting powder and mix with 100 grams of petroleum jelly. However, if the lesion is wet and suppurating, it is better to mix the above powder with water and apply externally. When oil-based ointments are applied to damp hot, suppurating lesions, this can cause the dampness and heat to spread laterally through the skin results in further adjacent eruptions.

Si Huang Gao (Four Yellow Ointment)

Radix Et Rhizoma Rhei (*Da Huang*)
Cortex Phellodendri (*Huang Bai*)
Radix Scutellariae Baicalensis (*Huang Qin*)
Rhizoma Coptidis Chinensis (*Huang Lian*)

Take equal portions of these and grind into powder. To make a paste, take 20 grams of the above powder and mix with 80 grams of petroleum jelly. However, the same comment as made above applies here as well. If the lesions are wet and suppurating, it is better to use this powder mixed with water instead.

Another, very effective external application for an open, glistening, and wet herpes lesion is to mix a small bit of powdered Realgar (*Xiong Huang*) with rubbing alcohol. Mix into a orange paint and apply directly to the head of the open lesion being careful not to get on the surrounding, healthy skin. Repeat this 3-4 times per day. This will usually cause a dry scab to form over the lesion within 24 hours.

Genital Warts
Jian Rui Shi You

Yang Jian-bao also discusses genital or venereal warts in *Xing Bing Zheng Zhi (Venereal Disease Patterns & Treatments)*. Yang calls these *jian rui shi you*. *Jian rui* means sharp points. *Shi* means damp and *you* means warts. Warts are also called condylomata in Western medicine. The sharp points Yang speaks of are the acanthoses or spiky, gravelly protrusions on the heads of warts. Therefore, *jian rui shi you* is the modern Chinese translation of the Western medical term condyloma acuminata.

Yang begins by saying that warts are an eruption on the skin and superficial mucous membranes and are a proliferation of excessive matter. The TCM treatment of warts is first recorded in the *Nei Jing* chapter called *Jing Mai* or "Channels & Vessels". Later generations have called warts *qian ri chuang* (thousand day sores or lesions) and *ku jin jian* (withered sinew arrows). The founding ancestors of (our, *i.e.*, Chinese) national medical theory treated eruptions of warts around the anus and reproductive organs but rarely discussed these in the literature. The cause of warts around the anus and reproductive organs is dampness and moisture. In shape and color they are soft and pliable, dirty and filthy looking, and are very much like cauliflowers in their features. Therefore, present medical theory calls them *jian rui shi you,* while among the common people they are called *cai hua chuang* (cauliflower sores or lesions).

1. Etiology & Pathophysiology

The cause of genital warts is the human papilloma virus types I, II, and VI. These mainly infect the epithelial cells and their only host is humans. This disease mostly erupts around the external genitalia and anus. It does not merely invade and violate the skin but can also affect the mucous membranes. Currently it is believed that eruption of genital warts is perhaps related to cervical cancer.

This disease crosses the boundaries of both venereal and infectious diseases. The onset of this disease also has to do with faulty hygenic practices in its suffers and is related to unclean dampness in the affected area due to chronic strangury diseases (*i.e.*, gonorrhea), excessive leukorrhea in women, and an excessively long foreskin in men.

TCM holds that the onset of this disease is due to disharmony of the qi and blood and lack of meticulous hygiene plus unclean sexual intercourse giving rise to mutual wrestling of turbid and wind evils. These condense or congeal the flesh and skin and turn it (into warts). Or, (warts) may be caused by liver vacuity and dry blood causing the sinew qi not to flourish. (TCM believes that the genitalia are the reunion of the hundreds of sinews.)

2. Distinguishing Characteristics of this Condition

A. Latency period: 2-3 months

B. Affected Areas: Genital warts are commonly found at the boundaries of the skin and mucous membranes where it is damp and moist. In men, they mostly occur on the penile shaft, the ditch below the head of the penis, the glans penis, at the urethral opening, etc. In females, they mostly occur on the labia majora and minora, the area where the labia are tied together, the cervix, the vaginal orifice, on the perineum, and surrounding the anus.

C. Age: Older in men; more often younger in women

D. Lesions: Genital warts may occur singly, scattered about, or collected in a cluster. They may be greyish white or light red in color. The tumorous hyperplasia may be papilliform, cauliflower shaped, or coxcomb shaped. The main body of the wart may be large but the base may be narrow when seen from the outside. Its surface may be damp and moist and is soft and pliable. Because genital warts typically are found in secret places where they are constantly soaked, their form and color are filthy and dirty.

3. Treatment Methods

A. External Treatment Methods

Formula 1: Pound Fructus Bruceae Javanicae (*Ya Dan Zi*) into a mash and apply this paste to the affected area. Use adhesive tape to keep it firmly in place. Change this herbal medicine once every three days.

Formula 2: Use Folium Artemisiae Argyii (*Ai Ye*) to burn as moxa directly on the wart. Each day do one time. Stop when the wart sheds or drops off.

Formula 3:

Radix Isatidis Seu Baphicacanthi (*Ban Lan Gen*), 30g
Herba Equiseti Hiemalis (*Mu Zei Cao*), 30g
Rhizoma Cyperi Rotundi (*Xiang Fu*), 30g

Decoct in water and wash affected part.

Formula 4: If the external shape of the lesion obviously appears to have a stem, it is possible to tie a fine silk thread or hair around the wart's stem. After some days, the wart may spontaneously fall off or slough.

B. Surgery

If the lesion is large, it should be cut away or excised surgically. If the lesion is medium to small, it is possible to use a high frequency electric iron (*i.e.*, electrocautery), carbon dioxide laser therapy, or cryotherapy.

C. Internal Treatment Methods

Formula 1:

Herba Portulacae Oleraceae (*Ma Chi Xian*), 60g
Radix Isatidis Seu Baphicacanthi (*Ban Lan Gen*), 30g
Radix Lithospermi Seu Arnebiae (*Zi Cao*), 15g
Semen Coicis Lachryma-jobi (*Yi Yi Ren*), 20g
Folium Daqingye (*Da Qing Ye*), 30g
Radix Rubrus Paeoniae Lactiflorae (*Chi Shao*), 15g
Flos Carthami Tinctorii (*Hong Hua*), 15g

Decoct in water and administer internally, one *ji* per day. This formula is for predominant damp heat toxins.

Formula 2:

Semen Pruni Persicae (*Tao Ren*), 12g
Flos Carthami Tinctorii (*Hong Hua*), 15g
Radix Achyranthis Bidentatae (*Niu Xi*), 12g
Squama Manitis Pentadactylis (*Chuan Shan Jia*), 9g
Radix Rubrus Paeoniae Lactiflorae (*Chi Shao*), 15g
Cortex Radicis Moutan (*Dan Pi*), 12g
Concha Margaritiferae (*Zhen Zhu Mu*), 30g
Rhizoma Cyperi Rotundi (*Xiang Fu*), 12g

Decoct in water and administer internally, one *ji* per day. This formula is prohibited during pregnancy. This formula is for predominant blood stasis.

Inflammatory Conditions of the Cervix
Gong Jing Yan Zheng[10]

In *Shi Yong Zhong Xi Yi Jie He Fu Chan Ke Zheng Zhi (Practical, Proven Treatments in Integrated Chinese-Western Gynecology)*, the author, Guo Yuan, includes a section titled *gong jing yan zheng* under the chapter entitled *nu xing sheng zhi qi yan zheng* or inflammatory conditions of the female reproductive system. *Gong* means palace and refers the *zi gong* or fetal palace, *i.e.*, the uterus. *Jing* means neck. *Gong jing* literally means the neck of the uterus but is the Chinese name for the uterine cervix. *Yan* means inflammation. *Zheng* means condition. Thus, *gong jing yan zheng* means inflammatory conditions of the cervix or cervicitis. Because traditionally Chinese medical practitioners did not do pelvic exams or Pap smears, there was no traditional Chinese disease category which specifically related to the cervix. This category has been added to TCM due to the influence of modern Western medicine.

---

[10] The single most commonly seen cervical pathology in the West is mild to moderate cervical intraepithelial neoplasia or what used to be called cervical dysplasia. This condition is not dealt with in the Chinese medical literature for the simple reason that Chinese women are not routinely screened by Pap smears, the way one diagnoses cervical dysplasia. Typically, cervical dysplasia is clinically asymptomatic, just as is cervical cancer in its initial stage. Therefore, one should treat cervical dysplasia like the first stage of cervical cancer, with the understanding that liver depression qi stagnation as a pattern is typically complicated in real-life by a number of other disease mechanisms. If one identifies and treats for these using a combination of internally administered and externally applied Chinese medicinals and/or acupuncture, one can usually reverse mild and moderate dysplasia in three months.

Guo Yuan begins by stating that the cervix is the important threshold which prevents pathogens inside the vagina from entering the uterine cavity. However, the cervix itself is susceptible to invasion by various micro-organisms. Because inflammatory conditions of the cervix are often caused by inflammatory conditions of the uterus or uterine connective tissue, inflammatory conditions of the cervix itself are often overlooked. They are also often neglected because cervicitis tends to be mild.

Cases of acute cervicitis are often accompanied by congestion and swelling of the cervix and copious, purulent excreta. The common types of chronic cervical inflammatory condition seen in clinical practice include erosion or ectropion, hypertrophy, and Naboth's cyst.

Cervical Erosion or Ectropion
Gong Jing Mi Lan

The surface of the cervix is composed of squamous cells which live in a weak acid environment. When, due to various reasons, there is a change in the quantity or quality of the vaginal excreta and after prolonged immersion of the external portion of the cervix in such excreta, these squamous cells may soften and peel. This is especially the case if the excreta is alkaline in nature. After the squamous cells defoliate, columnar epithelial cells underneath extend to the exposed portion of the cervix. These cells are more used to living in an alkaline environment. Because these columnar cells are relatively thin and, therefore, the subepithelial vessels are more easily seen, the ulcerated area appears especially raw and red. This condition is called cervical erosion or ectropion.

1. Pathology

Simple ectropion: During the initial stage, the cervix is covered with but a single layer of columnar epithelium and the surface of the cervix is smooth. This is called simple ectropion.

Granular ectropion: In protracted cases, the epithelium proliferates and is accompanied by overgrowth of mesothelial cells. Because of this there appear numerous tiny granules. This is called granular ectropion.

Papillary ectropion: After even more time, the overgrowth of columnar cells is even more rampant and assumes the shape of a nipple or papilla. This is what is called papillary ectropion.

If this condition takes a turn for the better, either spontaneously or due to treatment, squamous cells displace the columnar cells on the surface of the lesion. This separates the columnar cells from the subepithelial tissues and leads to their necrosis and sloughing. When the cervix is again covered by squamous epithelial cells, this is deemed recovery of the ectropion. The normal line of demarcation between the squamous and columnar epthelial cells is close to the external os of the cervix. Sometimes this condition is confusing since old injury of the cervix can expose part of the cervical membrane which then looks similar to cervical ectropion.

2. Clinical Manifestations

The main symptom of cervical ectropion is increased *dai xia* which is mostly yellowish and sticky with a few cases being clear and continuous. As a result of irritation of the external genitalia due to this excessive *dai xia*, the genital area feels extremely uncomfortable. Cervical ectropion is also accompanied by low back soreness and bodily weariness and taxation.

Due to varied severity, clinically cervical ectropion is divided into three grades.

Grade 1 (mild): There is a smooth surface characteristic of simple ectropion. The affected area does not exceed 1/3 of the cervix.

Grade 2 (moderate): The affected area is more than 1/3 of the cervix but less than 1/2, or the affected area may not be extensive but is covered with papillary or granular ectropion.

Grade 3 (severe): The eroded area is more than 1/2 of the total cervix or less than 1/2 but covered with severe granular or papillary lesions.

3. Treatment

Although there are various approaches to the treatment of cervical ectropion, it is necessary to exclude the possibility of cancer. In terms of treatment, presently local treatment is most popular.

A. Applications to the Cervix

i. Chloro-prednisone powder: Take 50ml of powdered chloromycetin and 2.5ml of powdered prednisone. Grind these finely and dust the ectropionic surface.

ii. *Zhong Yao Zi Gong Wan* (Chinese Medicinal Uterine Pills): Place one pill on the cervix one time per week. Four such treatments constitute one course of therapy. This medicine should not be used three days before or after menstruation.

Prescription:

Alumen (*Ku Fan*), 585g
Resina Olibani (*Ru Xiang*), 10.5g
Resina Myrrhae (*Mo Yao*), 9g
Fructus Cnidii Monnieri (*She Chuang Zi*), 4.2g
Stalactitum (*Hua Ru Shi*), 13.2g
Realgar (*Xiong Huang*), 13.2g
Borax (*Peng Sha*), 1.2g
Sal Ammoniaci (*Nao Sha*), 1.05g
Acacia Catechu (*Er Cha*), 10.8g
Sanguis Draconis (*Xue Jie*), 7.5g

Minium (*Huang Dan*), 46.5g
Borneolum (*Bing Pian*), 1.05g
Secretio Moschi Moschiferi (*She Xiang*), 1.2g

Preparation: Boil the Alumen in two bowels of water until it looks thick. Add the first eight ingredients. Add 3-5 spoonfuls of water and cook for 10 more minutes. Then add the Minium and Dragon's Blood and two more spoonfuls of water. Wait until this boils and turns gelatinous before adding the Borneol and Musk. Stir well and add 30 milliliters of water. Use a mild fire to cook this into a paste. Pour this paste onto a stone plate, divide, and shape into pills of about 0.9 grams apiece. After 3-4 minutes, the pills will have cooled and dried and can be scraped from the stone plate for storage.

B. Electro-ironing Method

This method is indicated for the moderate and severe forms of cervical ectropion and is a relatively ideal method for treating cervical erosion at the present time. As a rule, one treatment will cure this condition. It is contraindicated during pregnancy or in those with other inflammatory conditions. Before applying the electro-ironing method, a Pap smear is necessary for excluding the possibility of cancer.

Prior to the procedure, first disinfect the vagina and cervix. The electric probe should contact the lower half of the cervix first followed by a back and forth, circular movement from the os to the border of the eroded area. Use this same method to iron the upper half. The pressure of the operator should be even and the entire eroded area should be covered. Otherwise the healing process will be adversely affected and can cause heavy bleeding when the scab falls off. If the cervical os is more eroded, the duration of the ironing should be longer and with greater pressure. The more the lesion extends to the periphery, the shorter the duration and the lighter the pressure.

After ironing, a 1% solution of gentian violet should be applied to the surface followed by dusting the area with furacillin powder. If a Naboth's cyst is found, it should be punctured first, the mucous cleaned away, and then the ironing can begin. During and/or after the operation, the patient may experience a sore, distended feeling in the lumbosacral area. No specific treatment for this is necessary. After the operation, the tissue may turn necrotic and fall off with a light yellowish, offensive, scorched smelling exudate.

After 7-10 days, this exudate may be tinged with blood or accompanied by a little bleeding. If this bleeding does not stop, hemostatic medicine should be administered and one should avoid vaginal examination. After about two weeks, the scab falls off and the wound is healed. During the healing process, personal hygiene is important and bathing in a tub, sex, vaginal examinations, and douching are all prohibited. Check-up should follow after one month. If there is still limited erosion, electro-ironing can be done after 3 months.

C. Electrocautery: Using a sparking electrocauterizer, one burns the eroded surface into a scorched, yellowish brown scab.

D. Fulguration: Treat the eroded area with a fulgurator to burn the surface.

E. Cryotherapy: This new method has become popular in recent years due to its relatively good results, low rate of recividism and complications, and shorter course of treatment. This method uses liquid nitrogen to freeze the tissues at *minus* 80-170° C via a probe. This process causes the cervical tissue to become necrotic and fall off thus resulting in generation of new epithelium and achievement of cure.

F. *Fu Zhi* Acidosodium liquid: Use a 1% solution of this liquid to rub the cervix three times. Follow this by pressing the eroded area with a cotton ball impregnated with a 20% solution of this liquid. Remove the cotton ball after 24 hours. Apply this liquid medicine the same way once every other day. This method is relatively quite effective for treating mild to moderate cervical ectropion.

G. Cone biopsy: In protracted cases of cervical ectropion, when Pap smear confirms the existence of dysplastic cells, or when cervical biopsy shows atypical overgrowth, cone biopsy is recommended.

Cervical Hypertrophy
Gong Jing Fei Da

Protracted irritation due to inflammation can make the uterine cervix hypertrophic and hard. This condition is often found in conjunction with cervical erosion. However, one may also see simple hypertrophy with a smooth surface. This condition is due to blood stasis and its treatment should be based on quickening the blood and transforming stasis.

Radix Angelicae Sinensis (*Dang Gui*), 15g
Radix Salviae Miltiorrhizae (*Dan Shen*), 15 g
Radix Rubrus Paeoniae Lactiflorae (*Chi Shao*), 15g
Caulis Milletiae Seu Spatholobi (*Ji Xue Teng*), 15g
Rhizoma Cyperi Rotundi (*Xiang Fu*), 9g
Radix Auklandia Lappae (*Mu Xiang*), 6g
Rhizoma Sparganii (*San Leng*), 6g
Rhizoma Curcumae Zedoariae (*E Zhu*), 6g

Decoct in water and administer internally.

In this formula, Dang Gui, Salvia, Red Peony, and Milletia quicken the blood and transform stasis. Zedoaria and Sparganium break stasis and scatter nodulations. Cyperus and Auklandia rectify the qi.

Cervical Polyps
Gong Jing Xi Rou

Due to chronic inflammation of the cervix, one or more variable-sized growths may form. These are crisp and fresh in nature and look like drops of blood. The size of such polyps is usually about that of a soy bean but can be as large as 5 x 3 x 3cm. This kind of growth is comprised of columnar cells and connective tissue. Immersed inflammatory cells can be found in the interstitial tissues. Cervical polyps are always accompanied by a certain amount of bleeding or hemorrhaging upon contact.

In the treatment of smaller polyps, curved hemostatic forceps can be used to chop off the polyp from its root. With larger polyps or with those with a thicker stem, surgery is necessary. In this case, the upper portion is chopped off with forceps followed by suturing to prevent bleeding.

Cervical Retention Cysts (a.k.a. Naboth's Cysts)

During some cases of cervicitis, the cervical gland and its surrounding tissues may become hypertrophic. When the gland is compressed by the surrounding connective tissue and becomes occluded, retention of excreta inside the gland occurs and gradually results in the formation of cysts of various sizes. Mostly the size of the cyst looks like that of a soybean with a circular, smooth surface and is hard in nature. Such cysts contain a mucousy substance. It is necessary to treat such cysts by puncturing them in order to expel the pus.

Acupuncture

In all of Guo Yuan's above discussions regarding cervical pathology, the emphasis has been more on modern Western medicine than on traditional Chinese medicine. Xia Zhi-ping, author of *Shi Yong Zhen Jiu Tui Na Zhi Liao Xue (A Study of Practical Acupuncture Moxibustion & Tuina Treatments)*, makes a bit more attempt to discuss cervical ectropion from the point of view of Chinese medicine. Xia says that this problem was traditionally discussed under the category *dai xia*. As for disease causes and disease mechanisms, Xia says that it is due to either damp heat pouring downward or vacuity weakness of the qi and blood. Xia also adds that, according to modern medical theory, it is commonly caused by childbirth, miscarriage, possible surgical injury to the cervix, staphylococcus, streptococcus, E. coli, and anaerobic bacillus infections. As for therapeutic principles, these Xia says are mainly to clear heat and disinhibit dampness. For this purpose, Xia recommends the following acupuncture-moxibustion formula:

Zhong Ji (CV 3)
Qi Xue (Ki 13)
San Yin Jiao (Sp 6)
Tai Chong (Liv 3)

This formula clears and disinhibits damp heat and regulates and rectifies the *chong* and *ren*. Using fine needles, puncture using even needling or draining technique. The needles should be retained for 30 minutes with intermittent stimulation. Treat one time per day, with 10 treatments equaling one course. For qi and blood vacuity weakness or kidney vacuity, add moxibustion at *Qi Hai* (CV 6) and *Guan Yuan* (CV 4). For spleen vacuity, moxa *Pi Shu* (Bl 20). It is also okay to use electro-acupuncture on the above points.

Cervical Cancer
Zi Gong Jing Ai

Returning to Guo Yuan's discussion of gynecological diseases, after the chapter on inflammatory conditions of the female reproductive system comes a chapter entitled *nu xing sheng zhi qi zhong liu* or tumors of the female reproductive system. Within this chapter is a section on *wai yin ai* or cancer of the external genitalia and *zi gong jing ai* or cancer of the uterine cervix. Under *wai yin ai*, Guo Yuan discusses only the surgical treatment of this disease and offers no TCM discussion at all of disease causes or mechanisms nor of any pattern discrimination. Under cervical cancer, however, Guo Yuan does include some information on the TCM treatment of this disease.

Most of Guo Yuan's discussion of cervical cancer is devoted to the Western medical pathophysiology, diagnosis, staging, and treatment of this disease. After all that, Guo Yuan says that in (China's) national medical theory, *i.e.*, TCM, cervical cancer was traditionally categorized under flooding and leaking and *dai xia* in terms of disease categorization. Most often, the TCM pattern categorization of this condition is damp heat and accumulated toxins. The clinical manifestations of this disease can include:

1. Bleeding: Vaginal bleeding before or after menstruation

2. *Dai xia* with various types of discharge depending upon the stage of the disease

3. Aching & pain: Lower abdominal pain may extend to the low back, the inside of the thigh, and even down to the lower extremity to the center of the foot.

4. Urinary system complaints: Pain with urination, frequent urination, possible hematuria, and, in advanced cases, anuria and uremia

5. Digestive system complaints: Primarily constipation but later loss of appetite

6. Lower extremity edema as the situation progresses

The Chinese herbal treatment of this disease is traditionally divided and discussed under flooding and leaking and *da xia*. TCM holds that cervical cancer is damp heat and accumulated toxins in the lower burner. Chinese medicinals can be used to treat this condition based on pattern discrimination along with the use of medicinals from the cancer-combating (*kang ai*) category. For instance:

Herba Oldenlandiae Diffusae (*Bai Hua She She Cao*): Clears heat and resolves toxins, disinhibits urination and disperses swellings, quickens the blood and stops pain

Radix Sophorae Subprostratae (*Shan Dou Gen*): Clears heat and resolves toxins, disperses swellings and stops pain

Semen Coicis Lachryma-jobi (*Yi Yi Ren*): Fortifies the spleen and disinhibits dampness, clears heat and discharges pus

Bulbus Cremastreae Seu Pleionis (*Shan Ci Gu*): Clears heat and resolves toxins, disperses swellings and scatters nodulations

Herba Crotolariae Sessiliflorae (*Ye Bai He*): Resolves toxins and combats cancer

Herba Scutellariae Barbatae (*Ban Zhi Lian*): Clears heat and resolves toxins, quickens the blood and dispels stasis, disperses swelling, stops pain, and combats cancer

Treatment Based on Pattern Discrimination[11]:

Liver Depression Qi Stagnation

This pattern is evidenced by emotional depression, chest and rib-side distention and pain, lower abdominal aching and pain, heart vexation, a dry mouth, and a bowstring pulse. Treatment should course the liver and resolve depression, clear heat and resolve toxins. The formula to use is

---

[11] The pattern discrimination below describes the progression of this disease. Most women begin with liver depression qi stagnation. This may be accompanied by a number of other related disease mechanisms, such as dampness, phlegm, blood stasis, spleen qi vacuity, depressive heat, etc. This first stage is where the cancer itself is clinically asymptomatic and is found by Pap smear alone. The second pattern describes the stage where the cancer has not been treated and now it has formed an ulcerous sore. The third pattern, liver-kidney yin vacuity, typically describes someone who has been ill with this disease for some time. Therefore, due to a combination of enduring disease and heroic treatment via chemotherapy and radiation, yin has become damaged and consumed and the patient is emaciated. The final pattern is the end stage of this disease. The cancer has metastasized to affect the function of a number of internal organs. Therefore, the patient is now qi and blood, yin and yang vacuous and depleted. This progression is a common and recurrent one in the pattern discrimination of all types of cancers.

Xiao Yao San Jia Jian (Rambling Powder with Additions & Subtractions).

Radix Angelicae Sinensis (*Dang Gui*), 9g
Radix Albus Paeoniae Lactiflorae (*Bai Shao*), 9g
Radix Bupleuri (*Chai Hu*), 9g
Sclerotium Poriae Cocos (*Fu Ling*), 15g
Rhizoma Atractylodis Macrocephalae (*Bai Zhu*), 15g
Rhizoma Cyperi Rotundi (*Xiang Fu*), 9g
Radix Linderae Strychnifoliae (*Wu Yao*), 9g
Herba Oldenlandiae Diffusae (*Bai Hua She She Cao*), 30g

Decoct in water and administer internally.

Xiao Yao San courses the liver and rectifies the qi. Lindera and Cyperus are added to strengthen qi-rectification. Oldenlandia and Bulbus Cremastrae Seu Pleionis (*Shan Ci Gu*) [*sic*] are added to clear heat and resolve toxins.[12]

Damp Heat, Accumulated Toxins

This pattern is evidenced by dirty, foul *dai xia* or *dai xia* like rice-washing water with offensive odor, aching and pain of the low back and abdomen, irregular vaginal bleeding, and a red tongue with thick, slimy, yellow fur. Treatment should clear heat and resolve toxins, fortify the spleen and transform dampness. The formula to use is *Pu Ju Ling Lian Tang* (Danadelion, Chrysanthemum, Smilax & Scutellaria Barbata Decoction).

Herba Taraxaci Mongolici Cum Radice (*Pu Gong Ying*), 30g

---

[12] This last set of additions is based on the idea that toxins play a part of all cancerous conditions. Therefore, even though there is no mention in the pattern name of toxins, if the disease diagnosis is cancer, then one should use some toxins-resolving medicinals from the cancer-combating category of Chinese medicinals.

Flos Chrysanthemi Indici (*Ye Ju Hua*), 15g
Flos Lonicerae Japonicae (*Jin Yin Hua*), 30g
Rhizoma Smilacis Glabrae (*Tu Fu Ling*), 30g
Herba Scutellariae Barbatae (*Ban Zhi Lian*), 30g
Semen Coicis Lachryma-jobi (*Yi Yi Ren*), 30g
Herba Artemisiae Capillaris (*Yin Chen Hao*), 30g

Within this formula, Dandelion, Chrysanthemum, Lonicera, and Scutellaria Barbata clear heat and resolve toxins. Smilax seeps dampness and disinhibits, urination, resolves toxins and clears heat. Coix and Capillaris seep dampness and disinhibit water and, therefore, clear damp heat from the lower burner.

Liver-Kidney Yin Vacuity

This pattern is evidenced by low back ache, upper back fatigue, vexatious heat in the five hearts, dizziness, tinnitus, a dry mouth, bound stools, vaginal bleeding, and a red tongue with scanty or peeled fur. Treatment should enrich the kidneys and nourish the liver, clear heat and resolves toxins. The formula to use is *Liu Wei Di Huang Tang Jia Wei* (Six Flavors Rehmannia Decoction with Added Flavors).

uncooked Radix Rehmanniae (*Sheng Di*), 12g
cooked Radix Rehmanniae (*Shu Di*), 12g
Radix Dioscoreae Oppositae (*Shan Yao*), 12g
Fructus Corni Officinalis (*Shan Zhu Yu*), 12g
Sclerotium Poriae Cocos (*Fu Ling*), 9g
Rhizoma Alismatis (*Ze Xie*), 9g
Cortex Radicis Moutan (*Dan Pi*), 9g
Herba Scutellariae Barbatae (*Ban Zhi Lian*), 30g
Radix Sophorae Subprostratae (*Shan Dou Gen*), 15g

Decoct in water and administer internally.

Liu Wei Di Huang Tang enriches and supplements the liver and kidneys. Scutellaria Barbata and Sophora Subprostrata clear heat and resolve toxins.

Spleen-Kidney Yang Vacuity

This pattern is evidenced by low back and knee soreness and weakness, counterflow chilling of the four extremities, lassitude of the spirit, dull comprehension, chilly lower abdominal pain, abdominal distention, loose stools, copious, thin *dai xia*, and vaginal bleeding. The pulse is sunken and fine. This pattern mostly describes patients in the later stages of cervical cancer with whom the most that can be done clinically is to mitigate their condition, alleviate some of their pain and suffering, and prolong their life. Treatment should mainly warm yang and supplement the kidneys. One should also use, to a lesser extent, heat-clearing, toxin-resolving medicinals. The formula to use is *Ba Zhen Tang Jia Jian* (Eight Pearls Decoction with Additions & Subtractions).

Radix Codonopsitis Pilosulae (*Dang Shen*), 15g
Radix Angelicae Sinensis (*Dang Gui*), 9g
Rhizoma Atractylodis Macrocephalae (*Bai Zhu*), 15g
Rhizoma Smilacis Glabrae (*Tu Fu Ling*), 15g
cooked Radix Rehmanniae (*Shu Di*), 15g
Radix Astragali Membranacei (*Huang Qi*), 30g
Rhizoma Corydalis Yanhusuo (*Yan Hu Suo*), 15g
Radix Auklandiae Lappae (*Mu Xiang*), 6g
Ramulus Loranthi Seu Visci (*Sang Ji Sheng*), 15g
Radix Dipsaci (*Xu Duan*), 15g
Fructus Evodiae Rutecarpae (*Wu Zhu Yu*), 9g
dry Rhizoma Zingiberis (*Gan Jiang*), 6g
Herba Scutellariae Barbatae (*Ban Zhi Lian*), 30g
Semen Coicis Lachryma-jobi (*Yi Yi Ren*), 30g

Decoct in water and administer internally.

Ba Zhen Tang supplements the qi and nourishes the blood. Astragalus is added to supplement the qi. Loranthus and Dipsacus are added to relax the low back pain. Corydalis and Auklandia's purpose is to rectify the qi, quicken the blood, and stop pain. Evodia warms the middle. And Scutellaria Barbata and Coix clear heat and resolve toxins.

External Chinese medicinal therapy should be used at the same time in order to disperse inflammation, get rid of putrefaction, and remove stagnation as well as to lengthen and extend longevity. The Shanxi Provincial Tumor Hospital uses three formulas for the topical treatment of cervical cancer. One should select an appropriate one from among these based on an understanding of the functions and indications of each formula's ingredients.

Formula No. 1

Fructus Bruceae Javanicae (*Ya Dan Zi*), 3g
Semen Strychnotis (*Ma Qian Zi*), 3g
uncooked Radix Lateralis Aconiti Carmichaeli (*Fu Zi*), 3g
Calomelas (*Qing Fen*), 3g
carbonized Fructus Pruni Mume (*Wu Mei*), 15g
Pollen Typhae (*Pu Huang*), 9g
Pulvis Indigonis (*Qing Dai*), 9g
Arsenolitum (*Xin Shi*), 6g
Sal Ammoniaci (*Nao Sha*), 6g
Borneolum (*Bing Pian*), 1.5g
Secretio Moschi Moschiferi (*She Xiang*), 3g

Grind into fine powder and use externally.

This formula is able to block, stop, and destroy tumor cell proliferation. It makes the tumor retreat, transform, and slough while it simultaneously stops bleeding and fights infection.

Formula No. 2

Sanguis Draconis (*Xue Jie*), 9g
Smithsonitum (*Lu Gan Shi*), 9g
Rhizoma Bletillae Striatae (*Bai Ji*), 9g
Gypsum Fibrosum (*Shi Gao*), 9g
Corium Elephanti (*Xiang Pi*), 9g[13]
Alumen (*Ku Fan*), 15g
Pulvis Indigonis (*Qing Dai*), 9g

Grind into powder and use.

This formula quickens the blood, engenders (new) flesh, and astringes.

Formula No. 3

Radix Scutellariae Baicalensis (*Huang Qin*), 15g
Rhizoma Coptidis Chinensis (*Huang Lian*), 15g
Cortex Phellodendri (*Huang Bai*), 15g
Radix Lithopspermi Seu Arnebiae (*Zi Cao*), 15g
Borax (*Peng Sha*), 30g
Alumen (*Ku Fan*), 30g
Borneolum (*Bing Pian*), 1.5g

Grind into powder and apply externally.

This formula is suitable for controlling infection.

---

[13] This ingredient is elephant skin. Since it come from an endangered species, this ingredient should be omitted even if it were obtainable.

Bibliography

Chinese Language

Bai Ling Fu Ke, Han Bai-ling, Heilongjiang People's Press, Harbin, 1983

Chang Jian Pi Fu Bing Zhong Yi Zhi Liao Jian Bian, Liang Jian-hui, People's Hygiene Press, Beijing, 1986

Cheng Tan An Zhen Jiu Xuan Ji, Cheng Tan-an, Shanghai Science & Technology Press, Shanghai, 1986

Fu Ke Bing, Bing Yin Lee *et al.*, California Certified Acupuncturists Association, Oakland, CA, 1988

Fu Ke Zheng Zhi, Sun Jiu-ling, Hebei People's Press, Hebei, 1983

Jian Ming Zhen Jiu Zhi Liao Xue, Zhang Gui-ling & Zhang Xiu-ji, Tianjin Science & Technology Press, Tianjin, 1986

Ling Yan Liang Fang Hui Bian, Tian Jian-lai, Chinese Ancient Book Press, Beijing, 1988

Nu Ke Mi Jue Da Quan, Chen Liang-fang, Beijing Daily Press, Beijing, 1989

Shi Yong Zhen Jiu Tui Na Zhi Liao Xue, Xia Zhi-ping, Shanghai College of TCM Press, Shanghai, 1990

Shi Yong Zhong Xi Yi Jie He Fu Chan Ke Zheng Zhi, Guo Yuan, Shanxi People's Press, Shanxi, 1984

Wan Min Fu Ren Ke, Mo Qian, Hubei Science & Technology Press, Hubei, 1984

Xing Bing Zheng Zhi, Yang Jian-bao, Chinese National Gynecology Press, Beijing, 1990

Yao Jiu Yan Fang Xuan, Sun Wen-qi & Zhun Jun-bo, China Books Press, Hong Kong, 1986

Yi Zong Jin Jian, Vol. 1 & 2, Wu Qian *et al.*, People's Hygiene Press, Beijing, 1985

Zhen Jiu Yi Xue Yan Ji, Tian Cong-huo, Science & Technology Publishing House, Beijing, 1985

Zhong Guo Zhen Jiu Chu Fang Xue, Xiao Shao-qing, Ningxia People's Press, Ningxia, 1986

Zhong Yi Fu Ke, Shi Cheng-han, People's Hygiene Press, Beijing, 1989

Zhong Yi Fu Ke Shou Ce, Song Guang-ji & Yu Xiao-zhen, Zhejiang Science & Technology Press, Hangzhou, 1985

English Language

A Barefoot Doctor's Manual, Cloudburst Press, Mayne Isle & Seattle, 1977

A Handbook of Traditional Chinese Gynecology, Zhejiang College of TCM, trans. by Zhang Ting-liang, Blue Poppy Press, 1987

A Practical Dictionary of Chinese Medicine, Nigel Wiseman & Feng Ye, Paradigm Publications, Brookline, MA, 1998

Chinese Herbal Medicine: Formulas & Strategies, Dan Bensky & Randall Barolet, Eastland Press, Seattle, 1990

Bibliography

Chinese Herbal Medicine: Materia Medica, Dan Bensky & Andrew Gamble, Eastland Press, Seattle, 1986

Chinese Materia Medica, Vol. 1-6, G.A. Stuart *et al.*, Southern Materials Center, Inc., Taipei, 1979

Concise Traditional Chinese Gynecology, Xia Gui-cheng *et al.*, Jiangsu Science & Technology Publishing House, Nanjing, 1988

English-Chinese Chinese-English Dictionary of Chinese Medicine, Nigel Wiseman, Hunan Science & Technology Press, Changsha, 1995

Oriental Materia Medica: A Concise Guide, Hong-yen Hsu, OHAI Press, Long Beach, CA, 1986

The Merck Manual of Diagnosis & Treatment, Robert Berkow, ed., Merck sharp & Dohme Research Laboratories, Rahway, NJ, 1987

Index

A Concise Study of Acupuncture-moxibustion 55, 56
A Handbook of Traditional Chinese Gynecology 136
A Study of Practical Acupuncture-moxibustion & Tuina Treatments 80, 83, 93
abdominal pain 10, 29, 31, 34, 56, 128, 132
abdominal pain at onset of menstruation 34
abnormal vaginal discharge v, 1, 27, 61
abscess 68, 97, 98
amenorrhea 56
Annotated Fine Formulas for Women 102
antibiotics 67, 69, 98
anuria 128
aperture pain 33
appetite, lack of 55

Ba Wei Di Huang Wan 65
Ba Zhen Tang 25, 26, 31, 132, 133
Ba Zhen Tang Jia Jian 132
Ba Zhen Yi Mu Wan 26
Bai Ling Fu Ke 33, 75, 135
Bai Ling's Gynecology 33, 75
Bai Shao Yao San 16
Bai Zheng Fu 92
Bao Ming Ji 92
Bao Yin Jian 17
bartholinitis 97-99
bedroom harm 33
Bensky & Barolet 31, 32
Bian Que 6
biopsy, cone 125
bleeding disorder, conjunction 66
boils 86, 99-101, 123
Bu Xin Tang 104
Bu Zhong Yi Qi Tang 14, 62, 64, 65

cancer, cervical 116, 119, 127, 128, 132, 133
cancer of the external genitalia 127
candida 67, 69, 78
cauliflower sores 115
cervicitis v, 51, 56, 119, 120, 126
cervix, inflammatory conditions of 119, 120
Chang Jian Pi Fu Bing Zhong Yi Zhi Liao Jian Bian 135
Chang Yong Xin Yi Liao Fa Shou Ce 58
Cheng Dan An Zhen Jiu Xuan Ji 49, 135
Chi Xiao Dou Dang Gui San 103
chill harm 33
chong and *ren* 34-37, 40-41, 48, 58, 80, 127
chong mai 1
clitoris 110
cold, fear of 73, 100
cone biopsy 125
constipation 100, 128
corticosteroids 67
cryotherapy 117, 124
cystitis 110

dai, clotty colored *hei* 41
dai mai v, 3, 4, 6, 8, 9, 11, 36, 37, 40, 41, 45, 46, 51, 53-58, 73, 80
dai, white 6, 7, 16, 26, 29, 34, 35, 39, 40, 50, 54-57, 64, 73, 81, 84, 91
dai xia v, 1, 3-7, 12-14, 16, 26, 27, 29-35, 37-42, 45-59, 61, 64, 73, 74, 76, 79, 81, 83, 85, 87, 91, 121, 126, 128, 130, 132
Dai Xia Douche 81
dai, yellow 6, 9, 21, 34, 35, 37, 56, 76, 86
dan tian 9, 10
Dao De Jing 61
diabetes 85
diarrhea 55, 56
digestive system complaints 128
disease mechanism 4, 5, 33, 73, 84
dizziness 71, 73, 85-87, 131
dribbling 16, 23, 27, 33, 34, 63, 90, 106
dribbling and dripping 23, 28, 90

eczema 84, 89, 95
electrocautery 117, 124
emotional fluctuations 4, 6
estrogen 67

139

external genitalia, inflammatory conditions of the 85, 97

feet, cold hands and 73
Fen Qing Yin 13, 16
fetal gate 34
fever 26, 42, 64, 99, 100, 106, 110, 111
fever and chills 26
food harm 34
fox misled condition 103
frigidity 65
Fu Fang Ba Wei Wan Jia Jian 47
Fu Ke Zheng Zhi 45, 66, 78, 135
Fu Qing Zhu Nu Ke 36
Fu Ren Da Quan Liang Fang 41
Fu Ren Liang Fang 102, 104
fu zhi acidosodium liquid 124
fulguration 124
fumigating 104
fungal hyphae 70

Gan Cao Xie Xin Tang 103
Gao Fa Jian 66
gardnerella 68
genital candidiasis 67, 88
genital warts 115-117
gentian violet 113, 123
greater vestibular gland 97-99
greenish discharge 6, 8
Gu Yin Jian 20
Gui Fu Di Huang Wan 65
Gui Pi Tang 25, 65, 66
Guo Yuan 97, 99, 102, 119, 120, 127, 128, 135
Gynecology for 10,000 People 13

Hai Zang 16
hands and feet, cold 73
headache 110
heart palpitations 51, 53, 71, 100
heavenly water 1, 2
hematuria 128
hernia, bald 63

herpes 68, 109-112, 114
herpes genitalia 109
hormone levels 71
HSV II 109
Hua Shi San 23
Huan Dai Tang 14
hymen 97

indigestion 56
infection in the reproductive organs 57
inflammatory conditions 97, 119-123, 127
insomnia 53
itching of the whole body 79

Jia Jian Xiao Yao San 24
Jia Wei Bu Shen Gu Jing Wan 41
Jia Wei Dai Xia Tang 48
Jia Wei Er Chen Tang 26, 32
Jia Wei Xiao Yao San 24, 64
Jia Yi Jing 91
Jian Ming Zhen Jiu Zhi Liao Xue 83, 91, 135
Jiao Zhu Fu Ren Liang Fang 102
Jie Du Zhi Dai Tang 43
Jin Gui Shen Qi Wan 65
Jin Gui Yao Lue v, 33, 66, 102

Ku Shen Wei Pi Jiu 79
Ku Shen Xi Fang 103

labia majora 97, 100, 110, 116
labia minora 83, 97
Lang Ya Tang 102, 104
Lao Zi 61
Lei Jing Tu Yi 54, 55, 57, 91, 92
Li Huo Tang 11, 22
Lin Chuang Jing Yan Fang 37, 40-43
Liu Jun Zi Tang 15
Liu Wei Di Huang Tang 131, 132
Liu Wei Di Huang Wan 16
lifegate fire 4, 35, 41, 46
Long Dan Xie Gan Tang 21, 38, 62, 63, 70, 77, 86, 112

Index

low back ache 131
low back pain 40, 51, 73, 133
lumbar soreness and pain 46
luteal phase 2
lymphadenitis 110

Ma Huang Tang 105
masturbation 49
menarche 1, 2
menstrual irregularity 24, 25, 54, 56
Mi Yuan Jian 18
midcycle 2
Mo Qian 13, 26, 135
mons veneris 110

Naboth's cyst 120, 124
Nei Jing 1, 115
nei ke 61
neoplasms 101
night sweats 42
Nu Ke Mi Jue Da Quan 4, 5, 7, 13, 26, 32, 135
Nu Ke Zheng Zhi Yue Ken 33

oral contraceptives 67
ovulation 2

pain & sweating as if gnawed by a worm 34
Pap smear 123, 125, 129
parasites 63, 64, 68, 75, 77-79, 84-86, 89, 92
parasitic erosion 76, 84
pelvic inflammatory disease 56, 110
polyuria 18, 41
postmenopausal women 67
pregnancy harm 34
prenatal essence 1, 3
procaine 95, 96
prolapsed uterus 63
Pu Ju Ling Lian Tang 130

qi harm 34
Qian Jin Fang 92
Qing Gan Zhi Ling Tang 12

Qing Re Jie Du Chu Shi Tang 78
Qing Re Li Shi Zhi Yang Fang 90
Qing Xin Lian Zi Yin 20

rashness 53
red *dai* 6, 11, 22, 35, 49, 51, 54, 56, 58
ren and *dai* 3, 55, 73, 86
ren and *du* 6
ren mai 3, 7, 9, 10, 33, 45, 46, 48, 53, 56, 57, 92
reproductive tract, inflammatory conditions of the female 97
retention cyst 98

scabies 79
senile vaginitis 67, 71-73
sexual harm 34
sexual indulgence 6
sexual taxation 5, 27
Shang Hai Yi Xue Yuen Zhen Jiu Xue 58
Shanxi Provincial Tumor Hospital 133
She Chuang Zi San 88
Shi Quan Da Bu Tang 26, 66
Shi Yong Zhen Jiu Tui Na Zhi Liao Xue 80, 83, 126, 135
Shou Pi Jian 13
Si Huang Gao 113
Si Jun Zi Tang 15, 25
Si Ling San 23
Si Wu Tang 25, 63, 64
Simple & Agreed Upon Treatments for Gynecological Conditions 33
sleep harm 33
Suo Jing Wan 18
syndrome of eyes, genitals, and juncture of the skin and (mucous) membranes 106

The Collected Essentials of Treatment 92
The Complete Secrets of Success in Gynecology 4
The Golden Mirror of Ancestral Medicine 38, 61

141

The Great Compendium of Fine Formulas for Women 41
The Illustrated Appendix to the Systematized Classic 54, 55, 91
The Merck Manual 67, 137
thirst 10, 20, 23, 36, 38, 76, 77, 100, 111, 112
thousand day sores 115
tian gui 1-3
tinnitus 71, 85, 87, 131
Traditional Chinese Gynecology 48, 83, 86, 89, 93, 99, 101, 136, 137
trichomonas 67, 68, 84, 89, 92
tumors 50, 57, 101, 127

uremia 128
urethral opening 116
urinary fistula 84
urinary system complaints 128
urinating, difficulty 54
urination, frequent 86, 128
urination, pain during 34
uterine bleeding 13, 17
uterine cervix 110, 119, 125, 127
uterus, prolapsed 63

vagina not straight 33
vagina, swollen 62
vaginal excreta 57, 120
vaginal flatulence 65
vaginal fluids 2, 3
vaginal itch 76, 78-81, 84, 85, 91
vaginal itching v, 63, 68, 75, 81, 83-86, 90, 92-94, 96
vaginal piles 65
vaginal secretions 3, 50
vaginal vestibule 97
vaginal yeast infection 110
vaginitis v, 51, 56, 61, 66-69, 71-73, 75, 78-81, 83, 84, 88-90
vaginitis, senile 67, 71-73
vertigo 71, 73
vision, blurred 87

vitamin B1 95
vulvar ulcer 102, 104, 106
vulvitis v, 99
Wan Dai Tang 36, 46
Wan Min Fu Ren Ke 13, 135
warts, genital 115-117
water needle 96
Wei Xi Wan 19
Wen Dai Tang 8
white looseness 12, 15, 35
white turbidity 12, 13, 16, 35, 54, 55
withered sinew arrows 115
Wu Ling San 23
Wu Mei Yin Chen Tang 68
Wu Qian 61, 63-66, 136

Xiao Yao San 9, 24, 62-65, 87, 130
Xing Bing Zheng Zhi 83, 88, 109, 115, 136
Xiong She Wan 69

yang ming 2
Yao Jiu Yan Fang Xuan 79, 136
yeast infection 67, 110
Yi Huang Tang 10, 21, 46
Yi Zhi Tang 12, 15
Yi Zong Jin Jian 38, 61-66, 78, 88, 136
Yin Liang Xue Zhi Dai Tang 42
Yin Qiao San 111

Zhen Jiu Da Cheng 54, 57
Zhi Bai Di Huang Wan 71, 74, 88
Zhi Bai Di Huang Wan Jia Jian 71
Zhi Bai Di Huang Wan Jia Wei 74, 88
Zhi Liao Hui Yao 92
Zhong Hua Zhen Jiu Xue 54, 58
Zhong Yao Zi Gong Wan 122
Zhong Yi Fu Ke 48, 52, 63, 64, 72-74, 83, 136

OTHER BOOKS ON CHINESE MEDICINE AVAILABLE FROM BLUE POPPY PRESS
3450 Penrose Place, Suite 110, Boulder, CO 80301
For ordering 1-800-487-9296 PH. 303\447-8372 FAX 303\245-8362

A NEW AMERICAN ACUPUNCTURE by Mark Seem, ISBN 0-936185-44-9

ACUPOINT POCKET REFERENCE ISBN 0-936185-93-7

ACUPUNCTURE AND MOXIBUSTION FORMULAS & TREATMENTS by Cheng Dan-an, trans. by Wu Ming, ISBN 0-936185-68-6

ACUTE ABDOMINAL SYNDROMES: Their Diagnosis & Treatment by Combined Chinese-Western Medicine by Alon Marcus, ISBN 0-936185-31-7

AGING & BLOOD STASIS: A New Approach to TCM Geriatrics by Yan De-xin, ISBN 0-936185-63-5

AIDS & ITS TREATMENT ACCORDING TO TRADITIONAL CHINESE MEDICINE by Huang Bing-shan, trans. by Fu-Di & Bob Flaws, ISBN 0-936185-28-7

BETTER BREAST HEALTH NATURALLY with CHINESE MEDICINE by Honora Lee Wolfe & Bob Flaws ISBN 0-936185-90-2

THE BOOK OF JOOK: Chinese Medicinal Porridges, An Alternative to the Typical Western Breakfast by B. Flaws, ISBN 0-936185-60-0

CHINESE MEDICAL PALMISTRY: Your Health in Your Hand by Zong Xiao-fan & Gary Liscum, ISBN 0-936185-64-3

CHINESE MEDICINAL TEAS: Simple, Proven, Folk Formulas for Common Diseases & Promoting Health by Zong Xiao-fan & Gary Liscum, ISBN 0-936185-76-7

CHINESE MEDICINAL WINES & ELIXIRS by Bob Flaws, ISBN 0-936185-58-9

CHINESE PEDIATRIC MASSAGE THERAPY: *A Parent's & Practitioner's Guide to the Prevention & Treatment of Childhood Illness* by Fan Ya-li, ISBN 0-936185-54-6

CHINESE SELF-MASSAGE THERAPY: The Easy Way to Health by Fan Ya-li ISBN 0-936185-74-0

A COMPENDIUM OF TCM PATTERNS & TREATMENTS by Bob Flaws & Daniel Finney, ISBN 0-936185-70-8

CURING ARTHRITIS NATURALLY WITH CHINESE MEDICINE by Douglas Frank & Bob Flaws ISBN 0-936185-87-2

CURING DEPRESSION NATURALLY WITH CHINESE MEDICINE by Rosa Schnyer & Bob Flaws ISBN 0-936185-94-5

CURING HAY FEVER NATURALLY WITH CHINESE MEDICINE by Bob Flaws, ISBN 0-936185-91-0

CURING HEADACHES NATURALLY WITH CHINESE MEDICINE, by Bob Flaws, ISBN 0-936185-95-3

CURING INSOMNIA NATURALLY WITH CHINESE MEDICINE by Bob Flaws ISBN 0-936185-85-6

CURING PMS NATURALLY WITH CHINESE MEDICINE by Bob Flaws ISBN 0-936185-85-6

THE DAO OF INCREASING LONGEVITY AND CONSERVING ONE'S LIFE by Anna Lin & Bob Flaws, ISBN 0-936185-24-4

THE DIVINE FARMER'S MATERIA MEDICA (*A Translation of the Shen Nong Ben Cao*) by Yang Shou-zhong ISBN 0-936185-96-1

THE DIVINELY RESPONDING CLASSIC: *A Translation of the Shen Ying Jing from Zhen Jiu Da Cheng*, trans. by Yang Shou-zhong & Liu Feng-ting ISBN 0-936185-55-4

DUI YAO: THE ART OF COMBINING CHINESE HERBAL MEDICINALS by Philippe Sionneau ISBN 0-936185-81-3

ENDOMETRIOSIS, INFERTILITY AND TRADITIONAL CHINESE MEDICINE: A Laywoman's Guide by Bob Flaws ISBN 0-936185-14-7

THE ESSENCE OF LIU FENG-WU'S GYNECOLOGY by Liu Feng-wu, translated by Yang Shou-zhong ISBN 0-936185-88-0

EXTRA TREATISES BASED ON INVESTIGATION & INQUIRY: *A Translation of Zhu Dan-xi's Ge Zhi Yu Lun*, by Yang Shou-zhong & Duan Wu-jin, ISBN 0-936185-53-8

FIRE IN THE VALLEY: TCM Diagnosis & Treatment of Vaginal Diseases ISBN 0-936185-25-2

FU QING-ZHU'S GYNECOLOGY trans. by Yang Shou-zhong and Liu Da-wei, ISBN 0-936185-35-X

FULFILLING THE ESSENCE: A *Handbook of Traditional & Contemporary Treatments for Female Infertility* by Bob Flaws, ISBN 0-936185-48-1

GOLDEN NEEDLE WANG LE-TING: A 20th Century Master's Approach to Acupuncture by Yu Hui-chan and Han Fu-ru, trans. by Shuai Xue-zhong,

A HANDBOOK OF TRADITIONAL CHINESE DERMATOLOGY by Liang Jian-hui, trans. by Zhang & Flaws, ISBN 0-936185-07-4

A HANDBOOK OF TRADITIONAL CHINESE GYNECOLOGY by Zhejiang College of TCM, trans. by Zhang Ting-liang, ISBN 0-936185-06-6 (4th edit.)

A HANDBOOK OF MENSTRUAL DISEASES IN CHINESE MEDICINE by Bob Flaws ISBN 0-936185-82-1

A HANDBOOK of TCM PEDIATRICS by Bob Flaws, ISBN 0-936185-72-4

A HANDBOOK OF TCM UROLOGY & MALE SEXUAL DYSFUNCTION by Anna Lin, OMD, ISBN 0-936185-36-8

THE HEART & ESSENCE OF DAN-XI'S METHODS OF TREATMENT by Xu Dan-xi, trans. by Yang, ISBN 0-926185-49-X

THE HEART TRANSMISSION OF MEDICINE by Liu Yi-ren, trans. by Yang Shou-zhong ISBN 0-936185-83-X

HIGHLIGHTS OF ANCIENT ACUPUNCTURE PRESCRIPTIONS trans. by Wolfe & Crescenz ISBN 0-936185-23-6

How to Have A HEALTHY PREGNANCY, HEALTHY BIRTH with Chinese Medicine by Honora Lee Wolfe, ISBN 0-936185-40-6

HOW TO WRITE A TCM HERBAL FORMULA: *A Logical Methodology for the Formulation & Administration of Chinese Herbal Medicine in Decoction* by Bob Flaws, ISBN 0-936185-49-X

IMPERIAL SECRETS OF HEALTH & LONGEVITY by Bob Flaws, ISBN 0-936185-51-1

KEEPING YOUR CHILD HEALTHY WITH CHINESE MEDICINE by Bob Flaws, ISBN 0-936185-71-6

THE LAKESIDE MASTER'S STUDY OF THE PULSE by Li Shi-zhen, trans. by Bob Flaws, ISBN 1-891845-01-2

Li Dong-yuan's TREATISE ON THE SPLEEN & STOMACH, *A Translation of the Pi Wei Lun* by Yang Shou-zhong & Li Jian-yong, ISBN 0-936185-41-4

LOW BACK PAIN: Care & Prevention with Chinese Medicine by Douglas Frank, ISBN 0-936185-66-X

MASTER HUA'S CLASSIC OF THE CENTRAL VISCERA by Hua Tuo, ISBN 0-936185-43-0

THE MEDICAL I CHING: *Oracle of the Healer Within* by Miki Shima, OMD, ISBN 0-936185-38-4

MANAGING MENOPAUSE NATURALLY with Chinese Medicine by Honora Lee Wolfe ISBN 0-936185-98-8

PAO ZHI: Introduction to Processing Chinese Medicinals to Enhance Their Therapeutic Effect, by Philippe Sionneau, ISBN 0-936185-62-1

PATH OF PREGNANCY, VOL. I, Gestational Disorders by Bob Flaws, ISBN 0-936185-39-2

PATH OF PREGNANCY, Vol. II, Postpartum Diseases by Bob Flaws. ISBN 0-936185-42-2

PEDIATRIC BRONCHITIS: Its Cause, Diagnosis & Treatment According to TCM trans. by Gao Yu-li and Bob Flaws, ISBN 0-936185-26-0

PRINCE WEN HUI'S COOK: Chinese Dietary Therapy by Bob Flaws & Honora Lee Wolfe, ISBN 0-912111-05-4, $12.95 (Published by Paradigm Press)

THE PULSE CLASSIC: A Translation of the *Mai Jing* by Wang Shu-he, trans. by Yang Shou-zhong ISBN 0-936185-75-9

RECENT TCM RESEARCH FROM CHINA, trans. by Charles Chace & Bob Flaws, ISBN 0-936185-56-2

THE SECRET OF CHINESE PULSE DIAGNOSIS by Bob Flaws, ISBN 0-936185-67-8

SEVENTY ESSENTIAL TCM FORMULAS FOR BEGINNERS by Bob Flaws, ISBN 0-936185-59-7

SHAOLIN SECRET FORMULAS for Treatment of External Injuries, by De Chan, ISBN 0-936185-08-2

STATEMENTS OF FACT IN TRADITIONAL CHINESE MEDICINE by Bob Flaws, ISBN 0-936185-52-X

STICKING TO THE POINT 1: A Rational Methodology for the Step by Step Formulation & Administration of an Acupuncture Treatment by Bob Flaws ISBN 0-936185-17-1

STICKING TO THE POINT 2: A Study of Acupuncture & Moxibustion Formulas and Strategies by Bob Flaws ISBN 0-936185-97-X

TEACH YOURSELF TO READ MODERN MEDICAL CHINESE by Bob Flaws, ISBN 0-936185-99-6

THE SYSTEMATIC CLASSIC OF ACUPUNCTURE & MOXIBUSTION (*Jia Yi Jing*) by Huang-fu Mi, trans. by Yang Shou-zhong & Charles Chace, ISBN 0-936185-29-5

THE TAO OF HEALTHY EATING ACCORDING TO CHINESE MEDICINE by Bob Flaws, ISBN 0-936185-92-9

THE TREATMENT OF DISEASE IN TCM, Vol I: Diseases of the Head & Face Including Mental/Emotional Disorders by Philippe Sionneau & Lü Gang, ISBN 0-936185-69-4

THE TREATMENT OF DISEASE IN TCM, Vol. II: Diseases of the Eyes, Ears, Nose, & Throat by Sionneau & Lü, ISBN 0-936185-69-4

THE TREATMENT OF DISEASE, VOL. III: Diseases of the Mouth, Lips, Tongue, Teeth & Gums, by Sionneau & Lü, ISBN 0-936185-79-1

THE TREATMENT OF DISEASE, VOL IV: Diseases of the Neck, Shoulders, Back, & Limbs, by Philippe Sionneau & Lü Gang, ISBN 0-936185-89-9

THE TREATMENT OF DISEASE, VOL V: Diseases of the Chest & Abdomen, by Philippe Sionneau & Lü Gang, ISBN 1-891845-02-0

THE TREATMENT OF EXTERNAL DISEASES WITH ACUPUNCTURE & MOXIBUSTION by Yan Cui-lan and Zhu Yun-long, ISBN 0-936185-80-5

A Handbook of Menstrual Diseases in Chinese Medicine

by Bob Flaws

Menstrual diseases or *yue jing bing* are the first and, in terms of contemporary Western practice, the most important of the four divisions of Chinese medical gynecology. They include early, late, and erratic menstruation, scanty and excessive menstruation, prolonged menstruation, breakthrough bleeding, amenorrhea, dysmenorrhea, flooding and leaking, plus a whole host of premenstrual, perimenstrual, and perimenopausal complaints. The majority of commonly seen Western gynecological complaints fall within this traditional Chinese category of diseases. In this book, you will find everything you need to know to diagnose and treat this important group of female diseases with Chinese medicine.

$59.95 US

Available from Blue Poppy Press.

❏ Yes! I'd like to order __ copy(ies) of *A Handbook of Menstrual Diseases in Chinese Medicine* by Bob Flaws
❏ *Check/money order enclosed* ❏ *Please charge my credit card*

Name

Address

City/State/Zip

Daytime Phone

Credit Card #

Expiration Date

Send to Blue Poppy Press 3450 Penrose Pl. Boulder, CO 80301
Or order toll free at 1-800-487-9296
or Fax your order to 303-245-8362

A Handbook of TCM Pediatrics

A Practitioner's Guide to Care and Treatment of Common Childhood Diseases

by Bob Flaws

This book is a clinical manual of Chinese medical pediatrics. It covers the disease causes and mechanisms, pattern discrimination, treatment principles, and Chinese herbal and acupuncture treatments of 46 of the most commonly encountered childhood diseases. These diseases are arranged in a longitudinal manner corresponding to the typical ages at which these conditions tend to occur. Also included are discussions of immunizations, antibiotics, and the primary importance of diet in keeping children healthy and well. This book is a must for any practitioner who wishes to treat children with Chinese medicine.

$49.95 US plus $7.25 shipping

Available from Blue Poppy Press.

❏ Yes! I'd like to order __ copy(ies) of
A Handbook of TCM Pediatrics
❏ *Check/money order enclosed* ❏ *Please charge my credit card*

Name

Address

City/State/Zip

Daytime Phone

Credit Card #

Expiration Date

Send to Blue Poppy Press 3450 Penrose Pl. Boulder, CO 80301
*Or order toll free at 1-800-487-9296
or Fax your order to 303-447-0740*

A Compendium of TCM Patterns & Treatments

by Bob Flaws & Daniel Finney

This book is a practical compendium of TCM patterns with their disease causes and mechanisms, signs and symptoms, treatment principles, guiding formulas, main modifications, and acupuncture treatments. It is meant for both the student and the clinical practitioner. The authors have included numerous patterns previously not described in the English language literature as well as many complex patterns which are commonly seen in real-life practice in the West. It also includes a symptom-sign index and a formula index for easy reference.

$29.95 US plus $6.25 shipping
Available from Blue Poppy Press.
❑ Yes! I'd like to order __ copy(ies) of *A Compendium of TCM Patterns and Treatments*
❑ *Check/money order enclosed* ❑ *Please charge my credit card*

Name

Address

City/State/Zip

Daytime Phone

Credit Card #

Expiration Date

Send to Blue Poppy Press 3450 Penrose Pl. Boulder, CO 80301
*Or order toll free at 1-800-487-9296
or Fax your order to 303-245-8362*

The Treatment of Disease in Chinese Medicine

by Philippe Sionneau
and Lu Gang

*Volume 1: Diseases of the Head & Face
Including Mental/Emotional Disorders
Volume 2: Diseases of the Eyes, Ears, Nose, & Throat
Volume 3: Diseases of the Mouth, Lips,
Tongue, Teeth & Gums
Vol. 4: Diseases of the Neck, Shoulders, Back, Limbs
Vol 5: Diseases of the Chest & Abdomen ($24.95)*
These books cover a wide range of diseases that were previously not discussed in English and gives comprehensive pattern breakdowns with both herbal and acupuncture/moxibustion formulas including modifications for specific symptoms. These books can improve your clinical success rate and offer new insight into symptoms that Western patients present every day.

Vols. 1-4 $21.95 US, Vol 5 $24.95
Available now from Blue Poppy Press
*Call **1-800-487-9296** or send a check for books plus shipping $4.95 for one book, $6.25 for two, or $7.75 for three titles.*

Yes! I'd like ❏Vol. 1 ❏Vol. 2 ❏Vol. 3 ❏Vol. 4 ❏Vol. 5
❏ Check/money order enclosed ❏ Please charge my credit card

Name
Address
City/State/Zip
Daytime Phone
Credit Card #　　　　　　　　　　　　Expiration Date

Send to Blue Poppy Press 3450 Penrose Pl. Boulder, CO 80301
Order toll free at 1-800-487-9296 or Fax your order to 303-447-0740